Nine-Yea

A Memoir

Trevor Jones

Copyright © 2024 Trevor Jones

ISBN: 978-1-917601-42-9

All rights reserved, including the right to reproduce this book, or portions thereof in any form. No part of this text may be reproduced, transmitted, downloaded, decompiled, reverse engineered, or stored, in any form or introduced into any information storage and retrieval system, in any form or by any means, whether electronic or mechanical without the express written permission of the author.

DEDICATION

My book is dedicated to my dear friend the late Liz Edmiston, actress, ballet dancer, the funniest girl on the block and a constant joy in everyone's lives. Sadly missed.

THANKS

I thank my loving parents and my close family who followed my theatrical career path through the thick and thin periods, particularly my late brother John Albert Jones and his wife Eunice.

To those who contributed tirelessly during the extremely high and harrowingly low periods, of my life I would like to thank, my dear agent Lesley Duff, Ian Good, Helen Watson, Jo Monro, Paul Van Der Weele, Sheila Mackintosh Greenwood, Joyce Rae, Tony Adams, Christine Adams, Sophie Louis Dann, Nic Colicos and Jane Cremer.

For their endless support encouraging me to complete this book are Lesley Duff, Rosie Ashe, Hugh Ross, Kate Dyson, Alexa Povah, Glynn Sweet, Gordon Griffin, Jill Nalder, Jae Alexander, John Baldeston, and Michael Vivienne.

My inspiration to write at all in the first place was Tim Everdon.

Cover design is by Tim McQuillen-Wright

CHAPTER ONE

Of all the great loves of my life, the stage has been the most enduring. I found my calling before I could even write my own name – when I was barely old enough for primary school, my big brother, John, would drag me along to his drama group with him, where I was made to take part in play readings if there were not enough voices to make up the numbers. It's funny because I was too young to play any of the roles; too young to read the words, let alone understand them, but it didn't matter. I'd been bitten by the bug.

As soon as I was old enough, I became a chorister at our local church, following in the footsteps of my dad, big brother, and two sisters. I suppose my involvement was due to an affinity for showing off – I loved performing and playing pretend, and I got a lot of attention standing up in the choir stalls looking angelic – plus, I knew I was good. Clearly, my dad's Welsh heritage had blessed us all with good pipes.

Most of my life was centred around the church when I was young. I was raised by an Edinburgh-born mother and Welsh-speaking, soldier-turned-postman father, and I was the youngest of four children. We lived in a big townhouse, but not big in the sense that we were well-off. No, just big enough to accommodate all of us. There were four kids, my mother and father, my Aunty Marion (my mother's sister), and my maternal grandparents living on top of each other, and every one of us was involved with the church in some shape or form.

It wasn't that we were particularly religious. In fact, I never really gave much thought to the religious aspect of it at all. Any sort of event in the town was orientated around the church – concerts, get-togethers, parties, bake sales, the lot. That's how I got started with amateur drama.

There also wasn't all that much else to do in such a small town as Crewe, in Cheshire. It was an industrial town – most people who lived there either worked in the British Rail works or in the Rolls-Royce factory. Aside from the factories, there were a few shops, a pub on every corner, and a couple of cinemas. There was also the Majestic Ballroom, a dance hall.

The church hall community stuff I had been performing in since I was a child was very much what any young person in those days would join in with. But the adult amateur group I was involved with as I grew up was always kept at bay from my mates – they considered such activity not the most macho thing to be involved with. Besides, they would never come to see me in a show and wouldn't understand my interest or passion in theatre. I was a straight boy to them, not a poofy actor, and I wanted them on my side – I didn't want to get ribbed. Their main interests, it seemed, apart from football, were going to the pub and spending time looking up girls' skirts as they danced at the Majestic. To them, anything else was rather a silly, pointless thing to do. As I look back now, those days trying to keep up with the lads and dating girls was light years away from what I wanted to do.

But we often went together with our then girlfriends to the Majestic for an evening out. Many top performers from the Liverpool and Manchester pop scenes came to strut their musical stuff on the comparatively tiny stage there. It was hard to believe that such a tiny town played host to some of the biggest names in the music industry at the time: Cilla Black, Gerry and the Pacemakers, Freddie and the Dreamers, even The Beatles.

Of course, any pop concert was very different from what I was used to with theatre performances where there was usually a gap between the huge stage curtain and the seated audience. At the Majestic you were close enough to touch the performers if you got to the front of the crowd. It was electric.

I watched as screaming girls clambered to touch even the clothes of people like Billy Fury who sexily slid on to the platform. I wanted to join in somehow; something in me that I didn't quite understand made me want to jump up and touch him too. But with a girl on my arm that night, I held back.

When The Beatles brought out their first record, *Love Me Do*, in 1962, we Majestic Ballroom-goers in Crewe already knew who they all were by name. The Fab Four performed there several times, well before their first record was ever released, so they were well-known in Crewe. One week, when The Beatles came to play, I was visiting my Aunty Marion in Kent. At the time I had a girlfriend called Ann who was a live wire, a great laugh, and gorgeous to boot, so it was good to have her on my arm at dances and nights out. She, and most of my mates, went to the gig, and when I got home, my mates couldn't wait to tell me all about what I missed.

"Hey Trev," one friend said, grinning over his pint in the pub as I sat down to join the group, "did you know that John Lennon shagged your girlfriend this week?"
The group erupted into laughter. They clearly thought this was hysterical, and assumed it would wind me up, so they were eying me for a reaction. I pretended I was completely furious at the thought of John Lennon stealing my girlfriend. But neither my reaction nor the story was real. Supposedly, Lennon and Ann did share a kiss and a lager, nothing more. But I had no interest in having sex with Ann myself anyway. At the time, I just thought I was a late bloomer. It would be another few years before I realised the truth about myself.

Buying The Beatles' first record and singing along to it in my little bedroom was an awesome experience. The Mersey Beat music period was an astounding thing to witness for us teenagers living locally. How could it be that there were boys we knew by name who had suddenly recorded and brought out a single record? When it went to number one in the charts that year it was particularly magic for us kids in Crewe. Those boys came from nowhere, just like us, and they took the world by storm. It was so exciting to witness their success right from the early stages. I began to feel there could be something more for me ahead, other than working in the wages office of a factory.

When we were both teenagers, my big brother, John, and I attended the same grammar school. Although John left long before I joined – he was 11 years older than me – he was still well-known in the school; his name was on endless achievement boards, so I still felt his presence. He was a tough act to follow: a popular pupil, an amazing all-round sports person, and captain of the football and cricket teams. He wasn't bad at tennis either. Athletic, charming, and handsome – he ticked all the boxes.

I wish I could say the same for myself. I was a bit chubby and not in the academic a-stream, to say the least. In fact, I was one of the bad boys, which is funny to think about now. I had no school record to be proud of; my attention span was awful. I would mess about in class, smoke behind the bike sheds with the other naughty boys and skip most sporting activities. So, I was elbowed from various school activities and branded a disruptive pupil. None of this did anything to help my education reach any kind of decent academic level.

Contrary to the opinions of the staff, I wasn't misbehaving just for the sake of it. I really struggled at school, yet not a single teacher could get to the root of the problem. I seemed unable to grasp anything to do with the English language – reading text out loud in class was particularly awful. It was so bad that my teachers presumed I was messing about, or just dim. I used to get detentions for trying to explain myself, or teachers would hold me up in front of the other kids as an example of being the wrong kind of pupil.

So, I left school early, under a cloud, with no qualifications. I only understood why I struggled so immensely some 25 years later, when I realised I was dyslexic. My agent Lesley Duff's actor son was having major problems in school, and his parents were called in to discuss the problem. Lesley told me they discovered he was dyslexic. I asked what that word was, and what it meant – I had never heard it before. When she explained the problem, I said: "well that's normal, that was the sort of thing I would see when I tried to read text".

Before I understood my condition, it caused me such embarrassment, particularly when, early on in my acting career, I used to go to auditions for two-line commercials in London. The casting team would hand you a piece of paper with all the information about the product they were selling, and a couple of lines to say, somewhere on the page. The letters would scramble together in a heap on the page, which meant that I would either read the stage directions or not get any words out at all. Even when I did land jobs in theatre, my difficulty reading was a source of great shame for me. I'd be in the green room with other actors before rehearsals, and someone would hand me a magazine and say, "Ooh! Read my stars for the week", and I would freeze, or pretend I wasn't arsed about astrology.

How I continued, as an actor, to learn scripts with large speeches or monologues was frankly a miracle. But I did, from Shakespeare to Sondheim. Reading music for musicals was somehow easier as I could follow the visual flow of the notes on the score sheet up and down, and learn the words by rote, as I did when I was a choirboy.

I still do battle with dyslexia. But as I recognise it now, I control it better and underline everything I must read out loud in strong yellow – it seems to help. Although I still have difficulty deciphering the label on a can of beans.

After leaving school early, while I continued living at home with my parents, I devoted most of my spare time to performing in endless amateur shows. Each role, no matter how small, fuelled the fire in my belly – I knew onstage was where I wanted to be, and I was always dreaming of a larger slice of the theatrical pie. Plus, hearing family friends, neighbours, and even people I didn't know talking about how good I was in whatever production they had seen really made me believe I had what it takes. I could make my dream a reality.

I landed a job locally in the Lyceum Theatre's workshop at weekends, helping to build the sets. The vast workshop was not attached to the back of the theatre block but was an old warehouse area rented nearby to construct each stage set. All we had to do on Saturday nights, under the watchful eye of the designer, was dismantle the set on stage after the play ended its run, and slowly carry the pieces over the road for storage into the workshop.

Some of these set flats (as they are called) were mighty heavy, so it usually took two of us to carry one of them. They had been built to last in solid canvas-covered wood, secured with several four-inch-long nails. They had to be sturdy as they were reconstructed into another set a week or so later – several licks of a different coloured paint could make a huge difference to disguise what was once a castle into a modern drawing room. That's theatre. And in those days, there was little, if any, modern materials, or technology to help.

When the set was struck from the stage and stored away, we, as a small army, would carry – or drag – the bits of new set from the warehouse across the road to the stage to be constructed. It was always an all-night business, and not a pleasant one in wintery weather. Late one Saturday evening, as I was midway across the road carrying a heavy chunk of staircase, I heard a familiar voice shouting, "Wher Hey! Jones-*eeee*, Jones-*eeeeee*!" accompanied by lots of blokey cheering.

I knew immediately who it was, and who he was with. Barney, my oldest mate, and two more who were heading home, via the back of the theatre, completely pissed after a night out. They had probably been at the Majestic, which wasn't far away. To begin with, I was mortified that they had seen me with the stage management crew, wearing my workshop paint-smeared gear. I braced myself for them sending me up, as they had done before, for hanging about with theatre people ("They're all poofs, Jones-*eeee*"). They knew I had spent a lot of time performing with amateur companies over the years which was something they always smirked at.

But surprisingly, they were kind of in awe of what I was doing, probably as it was a manual – and therefore manly – job, even if it was associated with poofy thesps. They ribbed me a little as they were pissed, but at the same time, they praised me for doing something so very different to them. My new role as a workshop assistant was far away from our usual Saturday nights out together, and I suddenly felt quite happy, relieved, and proud that they were sort of approving.

As the months went by, I knew this was the world I wanted to be part of, and so I began to drift away from the Majestic Saturday night brigade. It dawned on me that meeting these mates, whom I had grown up with, late on that Saturday evening was a good omen. It was easier to move towards a different life from then on.

I was a repertory theatre workshop worker for over a year and got to appear on stage as an extra more than once in various large cast plays with the professionals. It was such an exciting time for a budding actor, working in amateur productions some weeks, then working alongside true professionals in the workshop.

I was surprised one day to receive a message from Julian Oldfield, the resident artistic director, who asked if I would be interested in joining the company at the beginning of next season, as an assistant stage manager. I could not believe my ears. Out of the blue, I was asked to join these thespians without having had any professional schooling. You can guess my answer was a big fat "YES".
Looking back, I see how lucky I was – there's no way an aspiring actor could enter the profession that way these days. I know I'm fortunate to have been in the right spot at the right time to start my career.
My parents were not at all happy that I left the factory job with regular money for a much smaller theatre wage. But, after I left the local repertory theatre and they saw I was happily appearing in various professional productions around the country, they soon changed their minds.

Within a few years, I was playing leading roles in most of the major regional theatre companies in the UK; I appeared in two international films directed by Clive Donner and performed in several West End London theatres. At a young age, I had already achieved more than I had expected in this profession. Especially as I'd never officially attended a drama school, apart from weekly vocal lessons at the Royal Central School of Speech and Drama when I was earning enough money performing as Jesus in the West End musical *Godspell*.

It wasn't until I really began working as an actor in my early 20s that I realised I was different to my mates of a similar age. Of course, the word I would use now is gay, but when I was young, that word was never used, and it was certainly not in my vocabulary at the time. Especially having come from such a small, country town. It just wasn't something I had heard of. I suppose I felt I was somehow, let's say, 'artistic', but I still preferred the company of women. I wasn't particularly attracted to men when I was younger, and I had lovely-looking girlfriends, but mostly they were friends who were girls. I was so clueless about the concept of being gay, or what it meant, that I was completely oblivious to the stage manager at my first theatre job having what I later registered as an enormous crush on me. I just thought he was an extremely friendly guy. I was completely naive.

Of course, the more theatre jobs I landed, the more actors I met, and the more I grew up, the more I realised what it was to be gay. But as far as people outside of the world of theatre were concerned, if I didn't have a girlfriend, it was simply because I was a busy working actor always on the road and just waiting to find the right girl, nothing more. That's honestly what I heard relatives say about me. I had no intention of telling them otherwise. There was, however, one shocking moment for me that stopped me in my tracks, when I heard my dad shouting at the television saying that he hated that "bloody poof Ted Heath", who was then the Prime Minister. Was it an indication that my dad thought I too was a poof? Of course, he didn't think that about me but hearing him say the word warned me he was at least aware of such a person.

I had never really had a conversation with any friend about my sexual orientation, apart from a fellow named Christopher Timothy. We became friends when we filmed *Here We Go Round the Mulberry Bush* way back in 1968; we got on like a house on fire from the get-go. After the filming we kept in touch with letters or chats on the landline, as mobile phones were a thing of the future. He was married with two children, and he invited me to his home in the country to meet his wife and kids. I instantly felt a pang of worry. I had never given him any indication I was gay – what if he wouldn't want me, a gay man, to be in his home or be his friend? It's sad, isn't it, that that was my first thought. But when the invite came, I felt it my duty to tell him my truth. Thankfully, Christopher was delightful when I geared up the courage to tell him. He said, firmly but kindly, that of course it was no problem at all – he just wanted to be my friend. The relief I felt that day that this very straight guy wanted to be my mate was immense.

Christopher is the only person, friend, or family member that I have ever officially come out to; he is the only person I have ever looked in the eyes and revealed: "I am gay".

Although I wasn't flamboyant (if anything, I was probably rather reserved), I was clearly a gay man to my theatre workmates, who never questioned anything. It was the consensus amongst fellow actors in the know that if you were a young actor in theatre, without a girlfriend, then you must be gay. It was simply accepted as the norm.

CHAPTER TWO

In the late 70s, I was enjoying life as a single young actor in London, although most of my time was consumed by the theatre. I worked a lot in my early years and show business at the time was so very different to the life of an actor these days. There were endless auditions to prepare for, work generally was abundant, and there was a choice of parts to pursue. Most of my friends wrote endless letters to prospective employers or to directors they had either worked for before or had met at a party, asking for work. The letter writing was relentless, but fruitful. On more than one occasion I had two theatre jobs at the same time in different cities, as well as having jobs in London's West End, so I was doing well. How things have changed. How on earth the young actors today cope with finding or pursuing work is a mystery to me.

Paul Van Der Wheele, one of my best mates that I had worked with on a film called *Alfred the Great*, decided we should share a flat together (we were never lovers, just mates). Paul had many sexual encounters and was very successful on the gay scene, to put it politely. I was less rampant than he; I was only ever interested if I thought they had the potential to be Mr Right.

Paul was a film production accountant, so he worked abroad a lot, spending weeks, sometimes months, at a time in faraway cities I could only ever dream of visiting. He spent most of his time, during our London years, working and partying in New York – let's just say both business and pleasure were plentiful there.

As he was so much more hedonistic than I, Paul heard tell of a certain illness that had reared its head in America. It was peculiar in that it seemed to affect gay men, so they said. To be honest, I took little notice of these stories at the time. But then a few months later, Paul's boyfriend, an American airline steward, began calling into our flat after long-haul flights from the US. He too had more first-hand tales of this weird something that was spreading in New York.

I had many friends living in London, and if I wasn't working on tour, I would often visit several gay couples across the city. They too would occasionally mention this odd illness that young gay men were contracting in America. Still, it was a faraway problem, none of our concern, I had thought. It would hardly reach our shores, would it?

But as the months went by, Paul heard more and more information, tales of the symptoms of this illness from the Americans. Each story sent a shiver down my spine.

Paul was really a party-goer – quite the hedonist. He often persuaded me to drive him to some of the gay clubs in London. I was never a big drinker, and as I have grown older, I hardly drink much at all. But rather late on those Saturday nights, I drove us from our vast, five-bedroom flat in Paddington Green – which I had found thanks to Sir Cameron Mackintosh, long before he became one of the most successful men in theatreland – to a gay venue in the centre of London, totally out of my head on some strong liquor and a spliff. I was living dangerously, which was so unlike my usual self.

Even at the clubs in Soho, we heard what were intended as whispers, had the music not been so loud, of this 'gay illness', as it was being called; it was becoming an unavoidable topic, but still we knew little about it. We had heard of this thing called Kaposi's sarcoma: large skin marks, dark red in colour, and terribly obvious to the eye. But, once again, none of us knew anyone who had seen these marks themselves or knew anyone who had the illness. So, we carried on regardless. I had my acting work to look for, so spent most of my time auditioning for absolutely everything I could.

I had no idea what was heading my way.

**

In late 1981, the musical *Annie* was nearly at the end of its hugely successful run at Victoria Palace Theatre in London. Casting for a touring version was already underway, and I was engaged to play Rooster, the bad brother of the leading lady Miss Hannigan, who runs the orphanage. I was delighted to land the role – it was a fun character part to play, and the music fitted my singing range, too. Plus, it meant a complete year's work on the road in a hit touring production.

The first day's rehearsal was mostly an informal get-together for all the cast to meet one another. The director and musical director greeted each of us warmly as we trickled through the doors of the grand auditorium. As a group of eager-eyed actors began to form, I searched each face to try and work out who was playing what role. I did the same for most of my jobs – I was usually pretty spot on.

We'd been standing around chit-chatting for a while when I saw a side door open, and one more person walked into the auditorium.

Even from the back of the stalls that looked down towards the stage, where I was standing, I could tell he was strikingly handsome, and not very tall. He was wearing a grey sports jacket over a simple white shirt and jeans. He looked smart – every bit the 80s pin-up. He started to walk slowly, and sideways, along a row of seats to join the cast at the back of the auditorium. At this point I wasn't sure he was even in the cast; he could have been theatre staff for all I knew. He didn't seem as outgoing or confident as the other actors – he was moving quietly so as not to draw attention to himself. But he certainly had caught my eye.

I watched him as he made his way to the centre aisle, and I fell in love with him right there and then. I really did.

The rest of that first day was spent arranging rehearsal schedules and simply getting to familiarise ourselves with such a huge acting company. Although I found it hard to concentrate on anything, or anyone, else. I couldn't help stealing glances at the handsome stranger. I didn't speak to him, but he would smile shyly each time our eyes met.

When I was working, I wasn't usually on the hunt for a boyfriend. I often spent time performing in different cities, but I was simply there to do my job, not necessarily to try and find a man in each city. It wasn't my goal. Although I knew I would make an exception for the Handsome Stranger.

Rehearsals took several weeks to get the show up to scratch – it was a massive production to get right before we opened in Bristol. I barely spoke to the Handsome Stranger at all, apart from nodding good morning to each other, as everyone did. I was mainly called for rehearsals with the leading characters I was performing with, so our paths never really crossed much. But I clocked on to several other cast members nudging each other knowingly as our eye contact continued to flourish.

The cast and crew settled into digs across Bristol, and I had no idea if this boy I fancied was sharing a place with another cast member, or whether he would be in the market for a housemate. I was hardly going to pluck up the courage to ask him, seeing as I had only just learned his name (Robert – it suited him), and we had barely passed the wistful eye-contact stage. I was always more circumspect then, but I also wasn't certain if he even liked men. Many of us didn't feel able to be free with our sexuality back then, as we can now. Of course, a lot of the dancers were a bit more overtly camp, but even they weren't as open as they could be nowadays.

As expected, the show was a triumph in Bristol, and we all settled down to perform there for several weeks. In those days, large productions like *Annie* never toured weekly. Each venue chosen for the production was booked for several weeks at a time. So, as the show continued in Bristol, I began to make more friends within the company and, to my delight, I had even started to chat with Robert in the local pub near the stage door after a performance. But I was hardly ever in his company alone. We were always with a crowd of raucous theatre folk, so trying to talk to him privately was almost impossible. I'd ask him little questions when group conversations broke off, or if someone got up to go to the loo. Everyone could see that Robert and I fancied one another – there was much speculation about the two of us from not only the other gay members of the company but also the girls who often dropped embarrassingly unsubtle hints about us getting together. A group of us would be squashed around a booth or huddled on bar stools, and someone would say, "Oh Robert! There's space beside Trevor, why don't you come and sit beside him", to which Robert would respond by turning an adorable shade of crimson. To make matters worse, his almost crippling shyness seemed to rub off on me – not that I was much of a smooth talker myself to begin with. He made me incredibly nervous. I was confident as an actor, yes, but not confident in my skills as a flirt, which meant we could barely get past small talk.

Robert also seemed to disappear most weekends, which threw another spanner in the works. After a few weeks of him slipping off, I asked a castmate where on earth he was off to.
"Oh, he's got a boyfriend in London," they said, "didn't you know?"
I'm sure the visible disappointment on my face betrayed my ignorance. I was completely crushed. I didn't know how serious the relationship was, and to tell the truth, I didn't really want to find out.

It was weeks before I worked up the courage to talk to Robert alone. It was a Saturday in early spring, and I had just come off stage. I saw him, standing outside the dressing room, looking rather awkward. I guessed that he was waiting for the room to clear to change out of his costume. He had an almost debilitating phobia – he absolutely hated being naked in front of people. Gymnophobia, I think it's called. Quite an unfortunate fear for an actor to have, seeing as so much of the job required taking your kit off in quick changes backstage, often so close to the stage that the audience could nearly see you standing there in your pants.

Robert smiled as I walked towards him, and I took the unusually empty corridor as my chance. I felt like a lovestruck teenager, nervously twirling my hair with my index finger as I blurted out the question: "Would you like to come on a drive with me tomorrow?"

I knew we both had the day off.

"Yes, I'd like that," he responded with a grin while his cheeks burned, right on cue. I had to stifle a cheer.

Our first date was a trip to the beach in Weston-super-Mare. It was a euphoric feeling, driving along the coast with Robert with the radio blaring in my old, beat-up Ford Anglia. It was also rather refreshing to be away from the full company, who were oblivious to our romantic day out.

We chatted all the way. He may have been a little shy, but he had a wicked sense of humour, which meant we spent most of the day in fits of laughter. He had an adorable laugh, particularly when he heard something rude being said by one of the other gay boys in our company.

Although the sun was splitting the sky, early spring by the British coast is still practically glacial. We had to push against the wind that bit at our faces to walk along the beach, but we were too wrapped up in each other to care.

Fish and chips were the order of the day, of course. What trip to the seaside is complete without them? The town was almost empty, so we barely saw a soul, and the solitude was liberating. I wanted so desperately to hold his hand, or perhaps pluck up the courage to lean in for a kiss. But I wasn't bold enough. As quiet as it was, it still felt risky to show too much affection in public – you never knew who would be watching. Even in London, gay men didn't hold hands in the street. I often wonder if we really appreciate how fortunate we are to be able to do that at all nowadays.

As the sun fell lower in the sky, just before we headed back to Bristol, I suggested we spend the night together. But sadly, neither of us could accommodate the other in our old-fashioned theatre digs. Plus, Robert still had his boyfriend down in London, and he was a perfect gentleman. We would have to wait for some time to be alone together in that way, but I knew from that moment that I would wait as long as I had to for him.

CHAPTER THREE

For the entirety of 1982, I was working alongside Robert in the *Annie* touring company. Although he and I spent our social life – along with other company members – together during this tour, we never seemed to stay in the same digs locations as each other. We were by no means an official couple either, as he still had a boyfriend back in London, so he was not a totally single young man. My courting days with Robert were a very old-fashioned affair compared to today's standards, so our romance was a slow burning one, to say the least.

As that *Annie* tour was coming to an end, I began to worry about what lay ahead of me. After spending a year on the road with Robert, it was excruciating to think that our paths may never cross again. Would Robert choose to go back to the London life he knew before and never see me again, or would things change? I had no idea what was on the cards for us. We never spoke about the possibility of continuing our relationship. Consequently, the end of the tour seemed to be the probable end of any kind of future together.

The tour was to end in Nottingham, and I was offered my next job in the same city at the other permanent theatre there. The rehearsals for the new job overlapped the last two weeks of the *Annie* tour, so I stayed in Nottingham when most of the cast and crew of the touring company headed for London.

That first week alone in a new city, rehearsing a new show and missing Robert, who was now back in London, was so painful. I was desperately lonely and lovesick, completely heartbroken at the thought of never seeing him again. But low and behold, there was a light at the end of the tunnel.

On Friday night I had a message from the stage door man telling me I had a visitor waiting there. To my surprise, I found Robert standing nervously at the door, waiting for me. He had travelled back to Nottingham, totally unannounced, to be with me. He said he had to finally finish with the London boyfriend before he could commit himself to me.

It had taken a year of gentlemanly courtship for Robert and I to finally get together as a couple, in 1983. It was a new beginning for us.

I had bought a lovely apartment in Tooting and was happy living there alone, so when the Nottingham job finally came to an end I went home. Robert and I had, by now, become an item, but he was still in a bedsit in Finsbury Park, a long way from my flat in Tooting. It was, quite frankly, ghastly. But to give Robert his due, he made the best of it. He was quite the homemaker. He covered the hideous walls with ten- by eight-inch photographs of famous theatre folk that he had taken. Not taken in the sense of pointing the camera – taken in the sense of keeping them for himself. When he was 16 years old, he became an office boy at H.M. Tennent's in Shaftesbury Avenue (which was the biggest impresario of the day). He was asked to clear out and throw away piles and boxes of photos of famous actors. There were production shots onstage of people like Noel Coward, Maggie Smith, Dame Edith Evans, and studio work of Cecil Beaton – the list was endless. He kept hundreds in his room in Finsbury Park. It was like being in a theatre dressing room, only not as pleasant.

As we became more of an item, we took the leap and decided that I could sell my flat and use part of the money as a deposit for a house that Robert and I could buy together. In some ways, it was a big decision, of course. I had lived with a boyfriend before, years previously, but we split up as, let's just say, he wasn't as committed to monogamy as I was. So, naturally, a part of me was cautious when things started getting more serious with Robert. That age-old fear of getting hurt again. But it's funny, at the same time, deciding to move in with Robert felt like the most natural thing in the world. I knew he was my soulmate, after all.

House-hunting was a long, time-consuming business, and as we were both auditioning for work at different times it was hard to arrange viewings. But I had a dear pianist friend who had a small, terraced house in Wimbledon, and I went to visit him there for singing lessons regularly. The size, shape, and location of his house was just what we were looking for, so our hunt was concentrated on the South Wimbledon area. We soon found a very similar house very near to my pianist friend, in an amazing location midway between two of the Wimbledon train and tube lines, so handy for getting into Central London for auditions and trips to the theatre.

We jumped at the chance, and quickly sold my flat so we could move in together as soon as possible. We had such a brilliant time decorating our new home and buying furniture, we even managed to have fun fixing the dilapidated garden area. Once settled there, we both managed to get theatre work too, so life was very good. Idyllic, even.

Robert and I weren't part of the young, wild, and free crowd who went dancing in Heaven. We spent so much of our time working in theatre and our side jobs, and when we did have the time, we would host wonderful dinner parties in our new house. I suppose both of us were old souls, in a way. Growing up, I had been into pop music, particularly The Beatles of course, but Robert had always been a fan of opera. When we moved in together, as he was totally enthralled with the voice of Spanish tenor José Carreras, the house would be filled with his operatic arias. I believe he fancied him. Classical music and several West End musical shows boomed through the speakers of our turntables. So much so that 80s electronic pop like Duran Duran and Spandau Ballet passed us both by, which feels rather criminal to admit.

To family members of mine and Robert's, the details of our relationship were never questioned. Like I said, I never had the discussion with my family, I never told them outright that I was gay. But – back when I thought I fancied women – I also never talked about any of my girlfriends at the time with my parents, either. We never talked about love or relationships; we *certainly* never talked about sex.

I doubt my sexuality would even have crossed my parents' minds. A wilful ignorance, perhaps. But I wasn't outrageously camp or effeminate, neither was Robert. I suppose to them, we were just two nice young guys in the same industry who lived together, as so many others did.

I guess it was a little different with my siblings, perhaps they had their suspicions when I was younger; perhaps, as with my friends, they just assumed. I never felt that I was missing out on something by not telling my parents the whole truth; I never felt that I had to consciously hide who I was, either. I felt quite lucky, in a strange way. Lucky in the sense that I never had to risk rejection by having that discussion. Robert came everywhere with me, and my family adored him – he was even invited as my plus-one to the wedding of my niece, Jackie. The introduction was always simply, "This is Robert, we live together", and that was that. It might not have been the whole story, but it wasn't a lie, either.

We may not have been able to indulge in public displays of affection in the way a straight couple could, but we would never have dreamed of doing that. Behaving as a couple in public, outside of safe spaces, was sadly not a luxury afforded to any gay person at the time.

Those were happy days, living together in our house in Wimbledon. Everything seemed to be going right for us, and after a string of odd jobs, Robert was lucky to be asked to audition for a new musical for the West End – *Snoopy*, based on the cartoon, *Peanuts*. After several nerve-wracking auditions, he was asked to play the iconic role of Charlie Brown. Perfect casting said everyone who knew him. The cartoon character was so like the real Robert: a cute, wholesome-looking, sweet boy who wouldn't hurt a fly. The production was a great success and ran at the Duchess Theatre, London for a year from late 1983 to 1984.

When we weren't working, Robert and I did almost everything together. I thought of him as more than a lover or a life partner, I thought of him as a soulmate in the truest sense of the word. We shared so many wonderful memories together over the years, including some fabulous holidays, even as young, struggling actors.

I remember our first trip abroad together as clear as day. We took advantage of a quiet work period and decided to get as far from grey and dreary London as we could afford. It wasn't the height of summer when we decided to go but it didn't matter, we simply wanted to get away. We searched through glossy holiday brochures in our local travel agents until we spotted some apartments in Corfu that we liked the look of, near a secluded beach, and walking distance to two nearby tavernas. It was perfect, a definite step up from our first seaside getaway to Weston-super-Mare.

Our apartment was practically on the seafront, with a balcony facing the ocean. We couldn't wait to rush down to the sandy cove and swim in the tantalisingly blue water. We had chosen Greece because we wanted a holiday with lots of sun, little realising it was of course early spring there as it was in the UK. But it was certainly sunny enough for us to get a tan, which is all we cared about.

We spent our days lounging about on secluded rocky beaches, or exploring the island, and our nights at either of the two tavernas near our apartment, where we would gorge ourselves on the most deliciously fresh seafood we had ever eaten.
This was the first time in our lives that we both ate crispy, battered calamari, and we loved it. Oddly enough, we had witnessed an octopus being caught earlier in the day on our shoreline by two little boys from the taverna, never realising that it would be our evening meal. Delicious.

As we sat eating our evening meal, we were regularly aware of floodlights sweeping across the sea from what we thought was a different island. We asked our taverna owner why it was happening, and he explained that the lights were from Albania, not from a Greek island. In those days it was not as free a country as Greece and residents regularly tried to swim the small strip of sea to Corfu. Presumably the floodlights deterred anyone trying.

We both thought Greece would be rather barren in the baking sun, but the island at this time was adorned with spring flowers. They were everywhere. We hired scooters to whizz around on and found ourselves stopping constantly to take pictures of the blooms. We even started to collect and press certain species we had never seen before to bring back home with us. They might well have been weeds, but to us, they were a stunning reminder of a blissful time away.

Both of us were eager to find any trace of where Gerald Durrell the writer and his family had lived on the island. It became quite a quest for us to find the location of the house, and eventually we found a local fisherman with a small boat who said he would take us. We sailed very slowly past beautiful coastline and were shown what the fisherman said with pride was "the house of Durrell". In retrospect, I wasn't so sure it was the correct house we sailed past, but it looked stunning.

We returned to London fresh with vigour and a bit of a tan for our next jobs, whatever they would be. We were established enough that work did come our way regularly, but like most actors we had to pick up odd jobs for some extra cash – being a theatre actor isn't always the glamourous life people think it is. For some extra money between jobs, we started selling bits and bobs at car boot sales and antique markets across the town, scouring jumble sales and any house clearance sales we could find close by.

My banger of a Ford Anglia had long since packed in, so I bought an old Post Office van – not too dissimilar from the one my father used to drive when I was a boy – which was painted white with a red stripe down its side. Quite an unusual mode of transport, but I loved it, and we could fill it up with any sort of rubbish we could find to sell on. We did very well, and it was quite a fun way to spend our time.

CHAPTER FOUR

I had been performing in a production of *Narnia* based on the C.S. Lewis book *The Lion, the Witch and the Wardrobe*, and we had a successful run in London, so our director, Christopher Biggins, decided to set his sights further afield.

America. New York. The Big Apple!

My jaw hit the floor when I heard the news: the production was booked to perform in a small off-Broadway church called Christ & St Stephen's used for theatre productions. Most of the original London cast were going and the rest of the company would be played by New Yorkers.

I couldn't believe my luck. I had never been to that side of the Atlantic; I could barely contain my excitement. I had heard stories from my dear friend Paul years before, but nothing compares to seeing it for yourself. I remember that eye-popping moment, coming into the city for the first time in a yellow taxi, craning my neck upwards towards the skyscrapers that loomed overhead. Coming from a small town where there was nothing higher than three storeys, it was like nothing I had ever seen before.

I felt totally honoured to be a young working actor there. Not only were we in a wonderful production and getting huge acclaim from audiences and the press, but we also had the chance to see all the amazing sights of the city for the first time. It was dazzling, and I was extremely happy, but keeping in touch with Robert in Wimbledon was difficult. The only way to communicate was by writing letters, and seeing as we were both working crazy hours and international post took so long to arrive, we didn't speak very often on the phone as it was so expensive. How things have changed in that respect.

I felt truly content and so incredibly grateful that Robert and I were so happy in our home life, and in our careers in the late

80s – the theatre gods were smiling down on us, it seemed. But in between our happy moments, we experienced our first loss.

In 1987, Robert and I attended the funeral of an actor mate of ours, Geoffrey Burridge. He worked in piles of West End musicals; he was outrageously funny and brilliantly talented. His death was a mammoth shock. It was sobering, too – Geoffrey was the first guy I knew to die because of AIDS.

**

In 1988, Robert got what should have been a life-changing call from the London theatre producer Bill Kenwright. Bill had decided to mount a new full production of the now infamous *Blood Brothers* in the West End. Robert had played the part of Eddie, one of the twins who dies tragically at the end of the show, in a repertory run in Northampton a couple of years before. He was brilliant in it, of course, so Bill had to have him for the West End debut.

The production toured for a short while to get it up to top speed before its big London opening in 1988 at the Albery Theatre on Charing Cross Road. The show, starring Kiki Dee as the mother of the fateful twins, was an overnight success, and Robert, along with his twin brother actor Con O'Neill, appeared in various magazines, newspapers, and interviews on television.

After Robert's contract with *Blood Brothers* came to an end in 1989, he and I both had a well-deserved break in theatre jobs. It was around that time that we were asked by our friend, Ian Good, who was then working as a theatre director at the local Polka Children's Theatre in Wimbledon, if we were interested in helping out in the Polka Kitchen. This was a small café attached to the theatre where the audience of children and parents could get teas and cakes when visiting the theatre shows. We agreed that the three of us would run the café based on a one week on and two weeks off basis. As Ian and I were generally good cooks, and Robert was a terrific baker, we jumped in wholeheartedly. It kept us busy and made us a little extra money. Plus, it was walkable from our little house.

Robert went overboard creating three-tier sponge cakes of all flavours, plus pretty cupcakes of every colour for the children to eat, or occasionally throw across the café. We worked hard during our shift week and the kitchen in our little house in Wimbledon was awash in flour and icing sugar at all hours. Robert was unstoppable, constantly creating new cakes – I even found him baking halfway through the night on more than one occasion. He was baking so much that he even started to write his own cake recipe book. I still have it.

I cannot remember how many months we worked at the Polka Children's Theatre, but we had such fun creating together and enjoying the spoils of our labour. Eventually, all three of us started to get theatre work offers and we had to finally agree to disband our kitchen chores and move on. But the last huge event we catered for was the Polka Theatre staff Christmas party. This was going to be a dinner that they had never seen before.

Robert found an old Mrs Beeton's cookery book and designed an expansive dinner menu which sprawled over several courses. We bought three huge turkeys and all the trimmings, platters of starters, in-between courses, a whole table full of delicious desserts and, of course, a Christmas pudding to finish. But that wasn't all – Ian and Robert had decided that they themselves would be the evening's entertainment, so in between all these courses they would parade around the dining room, performing songs and jokes and poems. The evening was a triumph; a night to remember.

Just before we started our next theatre contracts, I suggested Robert and I should have a holiday together and refresh ourselves. We chose to go back to Greece.

We flew to the island of Corfu again and there we had to take a ferry to the small island of Paxos off the southernmost coast. It's covered with olive groves and has only about 120 kilometres of coastline made up of small coves awash with restaurants. The stone dwelling that we were to stay in had once been home to an olive grove worker, and it had only the most basic cooking, washing, and toilet facilities. It was the most simple and rustic place we had ever stayed in. We loved it. Sometimes the simplest things are the most enjoyable.

Once again, we decided to hire scooters to get about, which, this time, turned out to be a disaster. Robert had an accident on his, trying to negotiate the winding, rocky, dirt roads. I watched, horrified, as he flew over the handlebars and landed with an almighty thump on the ground. He groaned and clutched at his leg, which had been slashed open by the jagged dirt path under our feet. There was blood everywhere.

There were no shops or chemists nearby, so I bandaged him up as best I could with a little first-aid kit I had taken in my backpack. But the wound took ages to heal, so for the rest of the holiday, we decided that scooters were out. We spent our days on secluded beaches nearby instead. Robert loved to swim, and I loved to watch him. But as I gazed at him standing in the turquoise water, I felt a knot of worry twisting in my chest. I had a feeling that there was something not quite right with him. He was losing weight.

CHAPTER FIVE

After a few more brilliant roles – including a run of *The Sound of Music* – Robert went back to *Blood Brothers*, at Bill's request, in 1991.

Onstage, he was a triumph, as usual. But offstage, I couldn't shake the feeling that something was wrong. One day, during a matinee show, he started to feel peculiar, so he went to see his onstage mum, Joanna Munro, in her dressing room. Jo knew something wasn't right from the moment she saw his reflection in her vanity mirror. He was sheet white and barely able to stand.

"Jo, I am not feeling at all well," he said in his usual polite, gentle manner, clutching the door for support.

"Darling, tell me what symptoms you have, maybe you're coming down with a cold," said Jo, as she walked towards him and touched the back of her hand to his forehead.

"No, there is something really wrong with me," Robert said emphatically, his voice wobbling.

Jo, as a responsible lady who adored her stage son, said: "I'm going to call the company manager and ask if you can miss tonight's performance". Which she did, and so Robert was sent home that evening to rest, in the hopes he would be feeling better for the next evening's performance. Jo likely assumed he was suffering with actor's exhaustion, simply knackered after a string of performances. It happens to us all – usually after a day's rest you're ready to hit the stage again. In that moment, neither Joanna nor Robert knew that he would never return to The Phoenix Theatre.

Typical Robert, despite being sent home sick, got the tube and walked from the South Wimbledon station back to our house. He was never one to be a drama queen. As with any other problem he faced in life, he played it down. But as much as he tried to brush it off, as soon as I saw him, my earlier suspicions were confirmed. Something really wasn't right.

I suggested we get an emergency appointment with the doctor that day – you could do that back then – for some peace of mind, but the doctor's visible concern only caused me to panic further. He rushed Robert up to the Atkinson Morley in Wimbledon, not far from our house, which immediately sent alarm bells ringing in my head. This hospital mostly dealt with stroke patients; surely Robert hadn't had a stroke at 34 years of age? The doctors seemed bewildered at first, then they began scheduling scans to check for signs of a stroke at once, but when the results came back, we were stumped, and relieved. There was no evidence that he had had a stroke at all.

Still no closer to understanding what was happening, Robert was sent for further tests at St George's Hospital in Tooting. The doctors were almost certain that there was something wrong with his brain because he was still presenting symptoms of a stroke – he didn't appear to be in control of his movements, for one – so they took his blood to rule out any possible infections.

That was when he was given the devasting, soul-crushing news.

Robert arrived home from St George's alone. I didn't go with him that day, he insisted he was able to go by himself. When I heard his keys turn in the door, I rushed to the hallway to greet him. His expression was flat; his eyes seemed far away. He stood there, just looking at me for a moment before he said it:
"I'm sorry. I'm HIV positive."
Words failed me. He looked so helpless. I hugged him and told him that everything would be all right. Of course, I had no idea if it would be. But the last thing I wanted to do was frighten him more than he clearly was already with a hysterical reaction.

Truthfully, most of the details of that day are a blur. I suspect I've locked them away in a far corner of my brain, never to be revisited. But I do remember my first thought after the initial shock of the diagnosis. What on earth was I supposed to tell people?

The stigma around the virus was awful. At that time, it was a death sentence, there were no two ways about it. But as well as fearing death, those that suffered feared ruthless judgement from those around them. The shame was enough for gay men to suffer alone rather than face being disowned by their families, or risk losing their jobs because others feared they would catch it too.

The way in which the virus was written about in the press was obscene. The news was saturated with reports on HIV and AIDS. Stories and strange speculations concerning young men who were infected were rife.

It was a terrifying time to be a young gay man in London. By the early 90s, the virus had stolen the lives of so many across the city, particularly the West End. Robert and I weren't ignorant of what was happening by any means, but neither of us were clubgoers or party boys sleeping around – the misconception was that to get HIV you had to be rather slutty, or sleep with the wrong sort of people. We had no idea that it didn't discriminate; that anyone could get it. That all it took was sleeping with one infected person months, or even years, before. No one knew how long people were infected before symptoms appeared, either. The virus had been around for years, but still, we knew almost nothing.

We never once thought this plague would come knocking at our door. In fact, as we went into the 90s, we genuinely thought the illness would peter out, or there would be a cure or pill designed to obliterate it completely. I guess, looking back, we were very naive.

I had to be careful what I said to anyone. The theatre company were simply informed that Robert was recuperating after a strange, stroke-like illness, and no more questions were asked. But his parents knew the full truth. Robert was incredibly fortunate in that sense. His parents rarely left his side. They were quite a remarkable couple and accompanied me regularly to speak to specialists at the hospital. They loved him dearly and were full of support.

I hated lying to our friends about Robert's illness. But I was scared to tell them the truth. I was scared that people would point fingers at me and ask a million questions about my own health. The illness was shrouded in mystery and shame; no one understood it. And so, as always, ignorance led to fear. So, I lied on an almost daily basis to anyone who asked me about Robert's condition, to protect him, and divert fingers from pointing at myself.

Days became weeks with his condition worsening, and I continued to lie to friends, to the actors, and to all the management of the *Blood Brothers* company. It was horrible. I felt incredibly guilty. Especially as his colleagues were so kind and thoughtful – Bill Kenwright, the show's producer, called to say that he would like to send both of us away for a holiday to recoup. He even suggested that he would pay for him to go to a special clinic to get well. He took the wind out of my sails. I just couldn't face telling him the whole truth, not yet.

I had only been able to keep Joanna Munro, Robert's stage mum, in the dark for two weeks, until, finally, she said to me: "I'm coming over to see you at home, and I'm bringing Robert's friend, Dee".

I knew I had to tell them the truth. They were barely through the door before it exploded from me, the news I was keeping hidden from almost everyone. Jo and Dee had both seen what was happening with others in the West End shows; they were hearing of more cases like ours, of boys who dropped out of shows due to an unexplained illness, never to return. It was sadly becoming increasingly common in theatreland. So, they knew. They just needed to hear it from the horse's mouth.

Jo was always on the ball – she was rarely faced with a problem she couldn't solve. So, after an ocean's worth of tears from the three of us, Jo and Dee told me that everyone at the theatre company – even though they didn't fully understand what was ailing Robert – wanted to create a benefit performance of the show for Robert, imagining that financial help would shoulder the burden as he recovered. I was beyond touched.

I had never heard of a West End theatre, as far as I knew, raising money for one of its artists. I knew that the boys in London shows who were infected by HIV and AIDS did get help from their own theatre family and their friends, but I believe that the benefit for Robert arranged by the complete cast and crew of the *Blood Brothers* company in August 1992 must have been possibly the first ever West End show to perform a complete midnight matinee show to raise money for one of its seriously ill actors. It was groundbreaking.

The CRUSAID Charity, which provided financial help for West End theatre performers, was formed in 1986. My friend Geoffrey Burridge, who died in 1987, had been the only person I knew well who had AIDS. He was certainly the first of my own set, of my generation, to have died. I had often wondered if Geoffrey was ever helped, in his last days, by that charity.

I was completely broken by Robert's diagnosis, but I was determined to be strong and positive for his sake. So, we traipsed between various departments in the hospital, often with his parents in tow, to find answers and solutions for his condition. He had volunteered to try various trial medications, desperate for a cure, but none of them were working, and he was only getting weaker.

Generally speaking, the nursing staff who, by then, understood this strange disease, were exemplary. But there was one specialist who was, for want of a better word, an arsehole. Robert was losing his speech, so his mum and dad and I went with him to a consultation with this doctor who either had no idea what he was doing or had made himself purposefully ignorant of the illness.

He started to ask Robert to say certain simple words, and he was barely able to get them out, when the awful man said: "How about, HIPPOPOTAMUS". I swear, he almost smirked as he said it. It was a ludicrous request. Robert was already visibly distressed, his parents were completely distraught, and I was completely fucking raging at how this so-called professional was treating a very ill young man.

I marched the three of us out of the consultation room as fast as I could. Thankfully, he was the only medic that behaved atrociously. Even if I could remember his name, I wouldn't write it down – he doesn't deserve the attention.

Eventually, Robert's condition got so bad that he couldn't walk by himself, so I had no alternative but to give up any hope of working myself. I couldn't leave him on his own, I needed to nurse him. I had no medical training of any sort, not even first aid. But I kept reminding myself that both my sisters were professional nurses in the hope that their natural calling to look after the sick would rub off on me. All I knew was that I had to keep him nourished, as well as clean and tidy, and try to keep his spirits up. I couldn't behave as if I was living with the fear of his death, which of course I was. I encouraged him, as best I could, to eat any food I could spoon-feed him; I administered any kind of medication that the doctors offered us, which at that time was azidothymidine antiretroviral (AZT). It was first prescribed in 1987, years after the first case of HIV was documented. We knew little of its success, it was still relatively new, and we had heard of its terrible side effects, but it was taken anyway – there was nothing else on the market.

There was an incredible HIV support group at St George's Hospital, and they supplied me with an amazing punk nurse from Germany called Heidi, who called in regularly, lifting my spirits by wearing her outrageous-looking clothes. She was the only person I relied on to monitor Robert's true condition.

Heidi and Robert had a special bond – they adored each other. Heidi continued to work with Robert on his speech by nattering with – or perhaps more like at – him. It was from Heidi that I learned what worried him most wasn't the inevitable that he was facing, it was leaving me on my own. For years we had looked after each other, just the two of us. He knew that he was no longer able to. His main concern was that I would be okay after he was gone.

Heidi was not only the best, most uplifting person to be around in the house, but she also helped me maintain a believable cover story by sharing any up-to-date information that I could disclose to anyone who asked too many questions.

I was busy all hours of the day looking after Robert at home, and since I wasn't able to work, I wasn't earning any money at all. I didn't even have time to take on any odd jobs on the side, as Robert and I used to do when money was tight. So, I tried to ask for some financial support via the benefit sections of the health service. I filled in forms as vast as *The New York Times*, but it seemed I did not qualify on any level, even though I was doing the work of several trained nursing staff and on call 24/7 in our house. I didn't get a penny from any government department.

I did, thankfully, have help from our closest actor friends who lived nearby. Ian Good and Helen Watson were regular visitors and hands-on helpers. They knew everything about Robert's condition. Once when Ian came with me to the hospital, he took me outside Robert's room and asked me directly what was really going on. I couldn't face lying to him, he was such a trouper for us both. The same happened with my fabulous agent, Lesley, and Helen. Wonderful Helen, who often cut Robert's hair (mine too) in our house when he was well and continued to do the same throughout his illness.

But no one asked me directly: "Does Robert have HIV?" No one said those three letters out loud. Honestly, I think people were afraid of hearing the truth, knowing what it meant for Robert. Or they were afraid of anyone they knew having the virus. To others who were in the know of what was happening to these young men, they didn't have to ask.

Where my strength came from to cope with our lives being invaded by this virus, I can't fathom, but I thank God that I had such wonderful friends to support me through this endless period of terrifying unknown. It was agreed by my support team that I could not nurse Robert 24/7, I had to at least have respite, some time for myself. So, once a week, on Wednesday afternoons, it was arranged that Heidi would look after Robert by herself and I would go swimming at the local pool in Wimbledon.

It was a bizarre feeling, knowing that for most hours of the day, I was on call, except for those few hours on a Wednesday. It was refreshing, a light distraction. As I cut through the water, my world seemed to be normal. It was a regular, fun thing to do – one of my favourite hobbies, ever since I was a boy. But I couldn't completely switch off. Each time I paused to come up for air, I was bombarded with thoughts about what would be waiting for me when I got home.

One day, around four months into my role as Robert's carer, I bumped into a fellow actor at the pool.
"My God! You look *amazing*," he said, his eyes bulging with astonishment, "you're obviously working out. You're *so* buffed up".
I was completely dumbfounded by his remarks. I felt totally exhausted, and I had no idea what I actually looked like – my appearance those days seemed irrelevant, I had bigger things to worry about.
"Oh well, you know actors, cutting back on all the cakes and sugar," I replied half-heartedly, before letting out a nervous laugh and awkwardly excusing myself from the conversation. Yet, when I caught my reflection in the changing room mirror, I realised my fellow actor had been right – I appeared to have changed shape physically. My chest, shoulders, and biceps indicated I was weightlifting. If my neighbour knew the real reason behind my toned physique, I'm sure he wouldn't have sounded so envious – it was simply due to carrying Robert around the house, up and down the stairs, and in and out of the bathroom multiple times a day for months.

Soon, Robert's condition became almost impossible to cope with. His body developed an involuntary twitch that propelled him around the bed in his sleep, which meant that nearly every night he would end up falling on to the floor. It was a terrifying spectacle to witness, especially as he was so incredibly frail. I was scared that he would hurt himself while I was asleep, so we decided that he should be hospitalised to see if they could help resolve this problem, and, at the same time, give me a break for a few days or, perhaps, weeks. As much as I hated being apart from him, I was relieved to have help. By that point, even with the support of Heidi and my friends, I was on my knees, physically and mentally.

Sadly, Robert continued to wriggle in the hospital bed and one day he flung himself on to the floor, striking his head on the bedside table on the way down. It was horrible. Worse still, this was the only movement he could really make. By then, he couldn't walk, even with help; he couldn't feed himself at all, he was totally spoon-fed. But the cruellest thing was he could no longer speak. His body was giving up bit by bit.

As his condition had no sign of improvement, it was the right time to tell Bill, on his next phone call, the complete truth. I had told him that Robert wouldn't be coming back, but Bill never lost hope that Robert would recover or be well enough to carry on as he once had. When I broke the awful news that Robert had AIDS, Bill was totally speechless for a while, and then all I could hear was sobbing on the other end of the line.

Robert's health continued to decline. The prognosis was grim. It was decided he should be taken to a hospice. There was no alternative. So, his parents and I agreed that he should be taken to a facility in our area, called St Raphael's.

Robert stayed there for only a few days. After nine years together, he died on 15th July 1992, with me, his parents, his sister, and his devoted friend Helen Watson by his bedside. Four days before his 36th birthday.

CHAPTER SIX

The morning Robert died, my dear friend, Helen, escorted me to register his death. I was in no fit state to go there alone – I collapsed on to the pavement outside St Raphael's Hospice. I could barely see through my tears; I could hardly walk. Grief consumed me. I was oblivious to the world that dared keep turning around me.

I couldn't tell you how we got to the registry office, it could have been in Wales for all I knew. I tried to focus on the registrar sitting behind the front desk, who had begun to ask questions. I was too busy crying to register what he looked like, but he was a middle-aged officious twat. Once Helen helped me to explain why we were there to the registrar he asked flatly, "Are you a family member?" without an ounce of sympathy.

"No," I said wearily, "I am his partner".

"You mean his business partner?" he replied curtly. His rudeness awoke me from my daze. In my distressed state, I said boldly: "No, I am his *lover*".

He was not impressed. In fact, he was visibly repulsed. But by now both Helen and I were enraged at his attitude. Going to register one's lover's death within an hour of them dying was bad enough, but to be questioned like that, with such ill-veiled judgement, was intolerable.

When we were questioned by the uncaring registrar about what he should list as the cause of Robert's death, there was a pause. Initially, neither Helen nor I had any intention of saying it was an AIDS-related illness. We presumed the registrar would have spontaneously combusted, should he have to write down anything so awful on his precious form.

"He died of PML," I said flatly, which was the abbreviated version, thinking he might understand. But he just scowled at me, looking perplexed and demanding more information. Then I remembered that just days before, Helen had helped me learn the full medical term for Robert's illness, which was quite a mouthful. So, the two of us said clearly, and rather slowly: "progressive multifocal leukoencephalopathy".

The registrar clearly couldn't believe his ears – by the looks of things he had never had to write such a word on any certificate. For me, it was important to get that right. Gay men I knew were not given the right to be open about their partner dying of such an illness. It was shoved under the carpet by so many people, including the families of young men who were infected with HIV and died as a result. I wanted this arsehole to know what my relationship was to this person who had died; I wanted him to know what had taken Robert from me. I didn't want it to be hidden.

The registrar clearly knew we were talking about AIDS – I could tell from the disdain on his face – but no one dies of AIDS itself. Surely, he must have come across other young men dying so unexpectedly in London by 1992. He glowered as he signed the certificate, and we left hurriedly.

Arriving home, my focus was to tell our loved ones the sad news. I rang my friend Paul who was working on a film set in Newcastle many miles away. He said he would leave immediately that morning and see me when he was back in Barnes, where he lived, later that afternoon. Several hours after having made many more calls to close friends and family, I pulled myself together to drive over to see my friend. It was a very tearful drive as all of me wanted to see Robert again rather than bother to drive my old car anywhere.

The journey from Wimbledon to Barnes took me alongside the entire length of Wimbledon Park, a beautiful area with endless wild woodland walks.

As I drove past there appeared to be an immense amount of flashing police vehicles. Dozens of them in fact and endless policemen walking everywhere.

For quite a moment my own grief was halted somewhat as I was astounded by the spectacle that was in front of me. What on earth had happened here?

Arriving at Paul's house I was greeted warmly, and I explained the commotion that I had driven past minutes before. He said he already heard there had been a violent murder on the Common this day. Then watching his television later, we heard the terrible news that a girl called Rachel Nickell had been murdered in daylight while her toddler son was nearby. An horrendous event never to be forgotten by me on 15th July.

The next hurdle was to engage an undertaker to pick Robert's body up as soon as possible from St Raphael's. Another heart-breaking task, as I soon realised that undertakers were not at all interested because of what was written on the death certificate. I found one eventually, after several failed attempts – there was just such a huge stigma about someone dying because of this strange disease. Could someone catch it after the person had died? Was it dangerous to touch that sort of dead body? They were medieval in their thinking, as though it was the Black Death. There were even local authorities in the UK who would disinfect the pavements near the houses of people who had died. Was it contagious in any form? Let's spray the roads just to be safe. Mental behaviour.

Arrangements had to be made for Robert's funeral. It was hard for me to handle – my head was all over the place. My friends were, once again, amazingly supportive. Dear Paul took a break from filming in Newcastle to be with me, and several of us sat around my dining table discussing what should happen and who had to be informed first. Robert's family were obviously completely grief-stricken. They wanted to be involved with the undertaker's arrangements, but they relied on my group of friends to mostly plan the service.

My mum and my family came down from Cheshire for the funeral. I was so deeply moved by the news that they would be attending. Although I shouldn't have been surprised. They adored Robert; he fitted in with them like he was part of the family.

The church chosen for the funeral service was St Mary's in Merton Park – a small, tucked away, Anglo-Saxon building. This attractive church had been frequented by Lord Nelson who attended services in the church with his lover Emma Hamilton, and he had bought a house nearby for the two of them to spend time in. To this day there is still a pew in Nelson's name, and his funerary hatchment still hangs in the church's roofline.

For me, my family, and Robert's family, it was perfectly acceptable to arrange a religious service here in St Mary's. I'd sung solos in churches as a child so choosing this venue was a perfect setting. Arrangements for Robert's service were made with a wonderfully helpful vicar who asked so many questions about Robert and our life together. This small act put me at ease – it was such a welcome change from the weird, often unpleasant, reaction from most people when they learned of how Robert died.

Sheila Mackintosh and Joyce Rae were theatre agents for both Robert and me. They were also great friends. Their office was up on Wimbledon hill, not very far from our house, which was handy. They insisted, well before most arrangements had been made, that they would, under their own volition, arrange a wake for after the funeral. They thought it fitting to engage the upstairs bar of Wimbledon Theatre, and arranged food and drinks for those attending the service to celebrate Robert's life. I was extremely thankful for their decision; it was amazingly kind.

The morning of the funeral I was at home alone, getting ready, slowly, when my dear friend Rosie Ashe arrived, much earlier than I had anticipated. Rosie had asked to sing at the service, and she informed me that she needed to use my living room for a full vocal warm-up before the funeral. I'm sure the arpeggios and operatic dexterity that filled my home on the early morning of Robert's funeral must have given the neighbours something to talk about. But Robert, being such an avid opera lover, would have been delighted to hear our dear friend's beautiful voice one last time.

I arrived at the church with Rosie to find it packed to capacity. The sight took my breath away. It was truly astounding to see so many people show up for Robert. I was so grateful that he was given such a fitting farewell. So many people had adored Robert, almost as much as I had – it was difficult not to love him.

The vicar spoke so kindly of Robert, and he made a point of addressing his final words of the service to me first, and then to Robert's parents. I realised later that this was because he was angry at all the hurdles I'd faced to give Robert a proper send-off.

Of course, the congregation was filled with thespians, who practically lifted the roof off when it came to singing the hymns. It was extraordinary.

Joanna, Robert's theatre mother, read H. Scott-Holland's poem *All is Well*; Rosie Ashe sang *Alleluia* from Mozart's *Exsultate, Jubilate*.

Con O'Neill, who played Robert's twin in *Blood Brothers*, gave a brilliant reading of Corinthians Chapter 13, 1-13. The words have always stuck with me:

Love is patient, love is kind. It does not envy, it does not boast, it is not proud. It does not dishonour others, it is not self-seeking, it is not easily angered, it keeps no record of wrongs. Love does not delight in evil but rejoices with the truth. It always protects, always trusts, always hopes, always perseveres. Love never fails.

At the end of the service, the brilliant vicar asked the congregation if we would all give Robert a final round of applause. The sound of all those hands clapping in that ancient church was deafening.

The news of Robert's death at the *Blood Brothers* company had hit them hard. Yet they decided, still, to continue with the benefit they had organised in his name. The Phoenix Theatre in Charing Cross Road at midnight on 4th August 1992 was packed to the rafters – people were even standing in the aisles as there were no empty seats, and there were queues in the street long after the last of the tickets had been sold.

Bill Kenwright, who was visibly shaken, gave a beautiful opening speech praising Robert's talent and wonderful, warm, honest personality. I was there standing with Lesley, my darling agent and friend, along with Robert's parents. It was a totally surreal moment for everyone watching the scene where Robert's character Eddie dies on the stage. There we were watching his replacement, Mark Hutchinson, die for him that night.

The evening raised around £17,000. Of course, had Robert lived, some of that money might have helped nurse him. But alas, I gave it to the Actors' Benevolent Fund instead, in the hope it could help others in our position.

The following year, in 1993, the stalwart cast of *Les Misérables* wanted to find a way to provide financial support for people living with the AIDS virus as the numbers continued to mount up. They arranged late-night cabaret shows in various venues all over London's West End to not only raise money for sick boys but to raise awareness of just how dreadful the deadly virus' impact had been.

The idea was then expanded by the forward-thinking *Les Mis* cast to include all the West End shows, one by one, that wanted to be on board and raise funds. Collectively, they formed West End Cares – which is now known as the Make A Difference Trust – an organisation that has gone on to raise millions of pounds for people, and families, affected by HIV and AIDS.

CHAPTER SEVEN

As the drama of Robert's death and the chaos of the funeral arrangements began to subside, I was, to say the least, decidedly low. There were days and weeks that I didn't know what to do with myself. I began to turn the house into a sort of photographic shrine to him. But a wall full of pictures didn't help relieve the sense of loss and bereavement, nor would they bring him back.

The grieving process affects everyone differently – there's no rules, no set pattern, no regulations on what anyone must do to feel better. I knew I had to get on with my life as best I could, so I tried hard to keep myself busy. Replying to the endless condolence letters took quite a while, which was good. I desperately wanted to keep up with Robert's dear family who were totally bereft, but yet still made the effort to see how I was doing.

But there were many moments in the evenings when I sat alone at my kitchen table and the desolation and loneliness would hit me hard. This particular evening, I didn't call my dearest mates to chat for a while. They had been so supportive, but I was scared I was becoming a burden to them. So instead, I poured myself a drink. And another. And another. You get the idea. I got completely pissed. I have said many times, I am not the world's biggest boozer, but a well-meaning pal had brought a bottle of whisky over the week before as a gift. At that moment, I didn't care if I wasn't a drinker, I was just desperate to numb the pain that I was feeling.

The local hospital HIV team had been such a rock when Robert was ill, and they told me, on countless occasions, that I should call them day or night if I needed to talk to someone. I had the number on a card stuck to the pretty fish tank in the kitchen that Robert and I had tended to so often.

That was the night to make the call. I dialled the number, but I was greeted with a recorded voice message that told me to leave a voicemail and that they'd call back. It seems they had an emergency problem of their own at headquarters. Great timing.

"Oh, for fuck's sake," I mumbled, semi-coherently, as I slammed the phone down. By this time, I was so stewed that I just decided to stagger up the stairs to bed.

Unbeknownst to me, while I was unconscious, the support team, clearly concerned, tried several times to call me back. Then, in the middle of the night, I was awakened by a deafening banging on my front door. I dragged myself out of bed, stumbled down the stairs, and opened the door, bleary-eyed and pretty out of it, to find three of the support team standing in my doorway, looking more than a little distressed. It seemed they had presumed, from my call for help and subsequent lack of response, that I had tried to harm myself, or perhaps even taken my own life. Clearly, they weren't going to leave until they heard signs of life.

I invited them in, rather embarrassed, and three of us sat around my kitchen table while one kind soul made me a coffee. We talked and talked through my anxiety and sorrow, and, as I came to with hot coffee in me, I began to feel terribly ashamed that I had put them through such trouble. What a tremendous team they were. But thankfully, they didn't have to visit again.

When I revisited sobriety, there was endless paperwork for me to fill in for the insurance on our house, the mortgage company, and Robert's bank. As Robert and I owned the house jointly there was no question from his family that the house was mine alone and they made no claim on it. I gave them full rein of any of his private things, and they were happy with that. But they insisted I keep his personal belongings at home if I wanted. I was lucky in that sense. This was a problem for a lot of gay men in my position whose families had refused to acknowledge the partner or their claim to any of the things they shared.

Robert's parents had always been accepting of me as his partner, which I know was an unusual situation. We heard of gay men who had HIV or AIDS being disowned by their families regularly through close friends of ours. But Robert's parents had always been good friends to me – we had even gone to France, just the four of us, when we knew he was unwell. They were lovely people.

As I was slowly coming to terms with the empty house, I thought it was time to look through Robert's wardrobe. I laughed out loud at one point when I found, in one of his coat pockets, two opened packets of ten cigarettes with a few missing. It seems he had secretly had the odd cigarette every now and then for years. He'd even hidden the stubs at the bottom of the packet. I had no idea. Cheeky so and so, I thought.

Then I found another surprise that Robert had hidden from me. There, in one jacket pocket, I came across several crumpled red tax demands. He had clearly not paid his tax for some time and had been getting reminders. I was completely oblivious. For all they knew he still owed this money. I felt sick to my stomach. Did that make me liable to pay the amount he owed?

It took me a while to muster enough courage to pick up the landline telephone, hands trembling, and ring the number on the page. When a well-spoken lady answered, I introduced myself and explained the dire situation I had found myself in. I could hardly breathe, aware that the result of this phone call could drastically alter my life.

I was clearly distressed as I relayed the ordeal, but she, caringly, told me to take my time. So, choking back sobs, I fully explained how he died – no point in avoiding the AIDS word by now, I thought. I told her that, for six months, I had been unable to work because I had spent almost every second of my day caring for Robert; I had not received any financial help from the government to cope with the situation, and I had no savings of my own – I was completely broke.

At this point, the unexpectedly kind, well-spoken lady cut in. "Please don't distress yourself any further," she said gently, "I am cancelling the demand. You will not have to sell your house or make any payments whatsoever."

I sat for a moment in silent disbelief. Then the tears resumed. I cried down the phone as I thanked her, over and over again.

Time began to pass again; it no longer stood still. Which was good, I suppose, although I was still angry at the buses that went by each day as though nothing had happened. My world had ended, and the buses were still running? Bastards.

A few weeks after Robert's death, I was offered a part in *Noises Off*, a rather complicated play by Michael Frayn in Manchester. I cannot fully articulate how splendid, how cathartic it was to tread the boards once again, and to be surrounded by actors who knew what hell I had gone through was like wrapping myself up in a warm blanket. Plus, the play was terrific. On stage, despite playing the role of someone else, I felt like myself again – you take on the mantle of someone else, and suddenly it's impossible to think about your own problems. You can't take your personal life on stage with you. But then the curtain would fall, I would go back to my digs, and remember that I couldn't call Robert for a chinwag at the end of the evening. I had never experienced his absence like this, ever. The loneliness was devastating.

I shared digs with an actress named Jenny Logan, who played my wife in the show. She became a dear friend, mostly because she was there for me in some of my darkest moments. One day, after rehearsals, when the loneliness set in again, I ran myself a bath, lowered myself into the steaming water, and began to sob uncontrollably. Jenny – along with the whole street, I'm sure – heard me breaking down, practically kicked the door down like she was armed police and I a fugitive, and insisted I get out so that she could console me properly. Actions like that are never forgotten.

It was the kindness of others and the love of my friends that helped me rise from the depths of my grief.

While I was in Manchester, I had decided that I wanted to find some way to commemorate Robert when I got back to London. I remembered he had performed in an open-air summer production of *A Midsummer Night's Dream* in the magnificent Cannizaro Park in Wimbledon, not far from our home. So, I decided to have a park bench made to be placed there in his name.

I asked for Robert's bench to be situated where the dressing room tents for actors would be placed for the next theatre season. Seeing it there in position made me very happy, and he would have loved it too.

My dear friend Helen and I often went for a wander in the park to look at the bench and reminisce. Then, luckily, in the following summer open-air theatre season I was asked to play Dr Van Helsing in a production of *Dracula*. During the run of the play, I was delighted seeing my fellow actors examine the bench with Robert's name carved on the back and hearing them ask: "who was this actor?" I was immensely proud.

The following spring, I felt it was an appropriate time to scatter Robert's ashes. I wanted to do it quietly on my own and thought it a great idea to let him have his last resting place on the stage area of the open-air theatre space in Cannizaro Park. To be honest, I had no idea if it was legal to do such a thing and, frankly, I never bothered to find out.

I chose a particularly cold, frosty February morning and arrived early wrapped up well, wearing heavy-duty leather boots to trudge through the park with the urn hidden under my coat. Once there, I wandered around to see if there were any maintenance gardeners about; luckily, as it was so wintery, there were very few.

Firstly, I concentrated on spreading him over the entirety of what would be the stage area in the summer season. Then, I decided to spread the remains of him around the circumference of the stage where I knew the dressing room tent areas would be erected. Mission complete, I left feeling surprisingly happy. No one saw me come or go.

I drove home with the empty urn beside me, only to find when I got to the front door and looked down to wipe my feet on the doormat, my frosted wet boots were covered in Robert's ash.

It may seem inappropriate, but I laughed my socks off as I looked at my now grey boots on my doorstep. He didn't want to leave.

**

After Robert died, I was encouraged to move on with my life by my dear friend, Ian, who, in the mid-90s, was manning Gay Switchboard, now one of the oldest LGBTQ+ telephone helplines, which provided help and advice to people worried about HIV and AIDS, in London.

"Switchboard staff have been given free passes to a new gay bar in town," Ian said one day, over a coffee (he made great coffee). He never went more than a few days without checking up on me. "Come with me?" he pleaded, "I'm going anyway, but I'd prefer not to be alone".

"Ian, I'm really not sure I'm ready for an evening out like that," I replied quietly, trying not to hurt his feelings. But he persisted – he clearly wanted to help me get past my housebound mourning stage.

"Look, it will cost us nothing you know. Switchboard volunteers like me are encouraged to go and promote the place." He eyed me expectantly.

I paused as I thought over what he said, sipping my coffee and trying to avoid his persuasive gaze.

"Come on let's go, let's have a laugh, you miserable so and so!" he begged. Which worked, he wore me down.

"Okay, fine," I relented, smiling at Ian's celebratory cheer in response.

He collected me a day or so later and we headed for an area of London I wasn't familiar with. The bar was heaving, and despite my reservations, and the fact that I was the designated driver, I managed to enjoy myself. I needn't have been surprised – Ian always knew how to make an evening fun.

It was exactly what the doctor ordered. I had shied away from social events for weeks. It felt good to finally be out of the house. I was beginning to feel human again. I was grateful Ian persisted.

Gradually, I began to venture outside more regularly. A day out by the seaside in Brighton was a regular trip in the summertime with friends like Ian. Fish and chips, a walk on the pier, and a beer were always welcome on those days by the sea. Luckily for us, our friend Paul had an extremely convenient little cottage by the station.

"We can stay over at Paul's place by the station this weekend," I'd say to Ian.

"Great, let's do it, I need a bit of sea air," Ian would eagerly agree.

Five summers well spent in Brighton passed by and, with each year, the thought of staying there permanently grew more appealing. There was nothing left for me at my home in Wimbledon, I knew that now. It was the home that Robert and I had made together, and, after all that time, it still didn't feel right to live there alone, without him. I had come to terms with the fact that it was time to move on.

I had always dreamt of living by the sea. For years, I had been quietly envious of my actor friends who lived in Brighton. It was still only a short distance from London, plus, houses were so much cheaper there than in Wimbledon. I knew Robert would have loved to live there, too – he was still in all my thoughts, of course. So, I decided a fresh start down on the coast was the way ahead.

My first Brighton property was a lovely Victorian house located quite centrally but up a hideously steep hill, which meant I would arrive home panting and red in the face. Not ideal (although it did give me exquisite-looking calves). I stayed there for a year, then decided to move to Saltdean, further out past the marina. It was a much quieter place to live, which suited me better, and there were gorgeous, detached houses with sizeable gardens that I could choose from. A gardener at heart, I always wanted to own a decent garden of my own, which isn't exactly feasible in London.

I purchased a three-bedroom bungalow which had a period spiral staircase in the middle of the hallway that led up to the third, en-suite bedroom in the attic. The garden I had yearned for was at the back of the house, with a vast 20-foot misshapen pond full of fish and pond life. It was my own little haven by the sea.

For a long time after Robert died, I lived as a single man. No housemates, no serious boyfriends, just me. Not because I wanted to be alone, but as a gay man I didn't find the dating game all that easy. Besides, it still felt too soon to contemplate that. The thought of trying to connect to another young man was simply not on the cards for quite some time, not that I was worried about the AIDS epidemic or trying to avoid anyone who I thought was not well. I just wasn't ready for dating.

There were so many gay bars and clubs in Brighton, it being the Gay Capital of the UK, all of which were wasted on me, I'm afraid. My disinterest in partying meant I had no desire to visit unless it was at the bequest of a friend, like Ian, when they came down for the weekend. He would say, "Let's pop in for a quick one" (it was never one), and I would happily go along for a drink with him – he was persistent, after all. But I never went alone. I was not at all active on the gay scene.

But as the 13th year after Robert's passing approached, in my lovely house by the sea, I began to contemplate the idea of meeting someone else. The traditional methods of gay dating weren't an option. Thank goodness for online dating! Not that it held a candle to what it is now. These days, the list of sites is comprehensive with endless choices, but in 2005, it was still a relatively new concept. The only gay site that I had ever heard of was one called Gaydar. I figured that if I wasn't going to hang around in bars, this internet search was the best way to meet someone, rather than waiting and hoping to meet someone I fancied at work.

When I opened the Gaydar pages, I headed for the foreign section almost instinctively – no chance of bumping into them in the local supermarket if things didn't work out. I also found talking to men from other countries much easier. I found them to be more polite than British men, to be honest.

Was it possible to find a new Mr Right, if I looked hard enough?
"Why not try your luck?" I said to myself.

CHAPTER EIGHT

Living by the shore helped me to heal. It was as though the sea air blew life back into me. And even walking by myself along the beach, I never really felt alone – I was accompanied by the rhythmic crashing of the waves, the sound of the gulls, even the occasional dog walker who said hello as I passed them. I could venture down a path beneath the famous white cliffs of the south coast – not far from my bungalow – along the beach, right across to Brighton on a sunny day. In the opposite direction, there was an under-cliff path that led to nowhere, a dead end. I discovered, by chance, that the acoustics in that sheltered area by the sea were terrific, which meant I had a free rehearsal space right on my doorstep. Before auditions, I would saunter along the beach beneath the spectacular cliffs and sing at the top of my lungs. I rarely saw another soul there, so it was the perfect spot. The only things to consider, when belting out a musical number, were a few bewildered seagulls.

In March 2005, I was offered a great role in a classic American musical called *How to Succeed in Business Without Really Trying*. It was to be staged in Chichester where I had worked on *Jesus Christ Superstar*, *Hollywood and Broadway*, and *The Government Inspector*, so I had fond memories of the city. The rehearsals were up in London for several weeks, then once the show opened in Chichester it was an easy car journey to the theatre from my house. What a lucky man was I working there again in a dream job.

The show was directed by a dear actor friend named Martin Duncan. He and I had been in a West End musical called *Happy as a Sandbag* years before, as well as various regional and London fringe productions. The choreographer at Chichester was another Brighton resident, the talented Stephen Mear. This amazing dancer had appeared in endless West End shows and won several outstanding awards in both London and on Broadway for his choreography. He was a theatre legend, and it was this much-admired man who, when my life was at a very low ebb, dragged me back into live theatre again.

Rehearsals of *How to Succeed* that first week were terrific – I had a decent role to play that suited me in this classy, old American musical. I was in my element, feeling very much alive and totally uplifted. I was back where I belonged.

At the weekends, I was at home resting, learning lines, and looking after my three cats. There was Dottie, an old black and white (the first cat that Robert and I rescued), Flossie, a fluffy grey beauty, and George, her son, a chunky black pussy (he was my favourite). My bungalow in Saltdean had three bedrooms, one of which I had converted into a study to house the thousands of records I had accumulated over the years. After dinner one evening in the early spring, I was sitting in my study, dwarfed by towering shelves of vinyl, browsing on my desktop PC – as I did in those days – when I decided to check in on Gaydar. A simple, black-and-white photograph caught my eye. It was of a handsome young man wearing a vertical ribbed sweater, standing in an almost empty street next to a car. From his picture I guessed he was mid-to-late-20s, not middle-aged like me; he looked Mediterranean – Italian, perhaps – and chic. I glanced down at the bottom of his profile to see his current location: Algeria.

I was intrigued.

As I read his profile, I realised I had no idea where Algeria was. I knew nothing about North Africa at all really, which was surprising as I had been rather good at geography at school. So, I rummaged around for my huge tome of a world atlas, from which I learned that Algeria is a rather large country on the edge of the Mediterranean Sea, with the Sahara Desert bordering it to the south, flanked by Morocco on one side, and Tunisia on the other. Miles away from me in England. No chance of any awkward encounters at Sainsbury's.

I lingered over this handsome fellow's profile. There was just something about him that drew me in. I had spoken with a few men on the site before, a couple from Scandinavian countries as I knew they spoke English well, but nothing ever came from those chats. This guy was different. He seemed charming. He had a gorgeous face – angelic, almost – which was lit up by an amazing, beaming smile. "Maybe he'll reply if I message him," I thought to myself, ruffling my hair absentmindedly as I do when I'm thinking.

I sent him one line: a simple, "Hello, you look nice". Not exactly an exciting chat-up line, I know. But frankly, I didn't think he'd get back to me. With so many men from all around the world using this, one of the only gay dating sites, the competition was fierce. There was no guarantee that he would reply even if I had thought of a stunning opening gambit, so I didn't want to waste my energy trying to flirt with a stranger. As soon as I sent the message, I switched off my computer. It was late, I was tired, and I had to be up early for rehearsals the next day in London, so I went to bed. But I was still thinking of the handsome Algerian, hoping he might see my profile photo and think I wasn't too bad a catch.

On Tuesday evening, after a particularly long and exhausting rehearsal in London, I slumped down in front of the computer in my study. It had been 48 hours since I made my move, so my hopes weren't high. I switched on the PC with a defeated sigh and suffered through the screeching drone of dial-up internet for one last look at my chances.
I sat forward with a bolt and felt a thrill race through me. A reply.
"I was surprised that I found a message from you in my inbox, thanks for that," he wrote, in perfect English. I actually felt myself blush.
"I really liked the look of you in that unusual picture," I responded. A bit pathetic, but my flirting skills were non-existent.
"I really liked the look of you too, that's why I'm replying." I smiled at the compliment.

We talked for hours over the next few days, asking endless questions about each other's lives, which were so different. There was much to discuss: where we lived, what our families were like, what we did for work, our favourite films (*Pride and Prejudice* for me; he was more into what film stars were wearing than their movies), and what kind of music we listened to (we bonded over our devotion to George Michael, and he sent me music videos of local Algerian and Lebanese singers; I enjoyed hearing these artistes but had no idea who they were).

He told me that he had studied English language at the University of Oran – to the initial dismay of his parents, who had hoped he might follow in the footsteps of his older brother, a doctor – but his true passion lay in the world of fashion and design. So, while he studied English at the university, he managed to secure a place at the only fashion school in the whole of Algeria, two courses at one time in the same city. Eventually, he was sent to Université Lumière Lyon in France, to finish the design course and receive his diploma there. He was a remarkably busy student, a hard worker indeed.

It was his dream, he said, to become a designer one day. After all, Yves Saint Laurent was born in Algeria. Why couldn't he follow in his footsteps? I smiled at his confidence.

He wanted to understand my world of theatre. An actor's working life in Chichester was difficult for him to wrap his head around, it being so alien to him, but he was extremely interested in the arts – after all, design and fashion play a huge role in theatreland.

When I tell anyone that I work as an actor, most people presume I am either famous, on television, rich, or all three. I was none of those things, but this didn't seem to faze him.

I asked him what language people spoke in Algeria; a tad mortified about my ignorance.
"I speak French and Arabic, like most people do here," he wrote, "and English of course. I often pick up bits of other

languages from simply hearing them, like Italian and bits of Spanish."

Impressive, I thought. He was gifted to be able to pick up languages so easily. I, like so many of my fellow countrymen, had not been blessed with that same gift. Although, three months before I first found his picture on the internet, I had started attending a weekly French language course nearby, in Hove. My friends had been curious as to why I was suddenly so keen to refresh my basic schoolboy knowledge. "Well," I had said, "I simply feel the need to familiarise myself with the language, in case I meet a gorgeous French man. You never know!"

How ironic that I should give up on the course only days before I did meet a gorgeous French-speaking man from Algeria. I kicked myself for not taking my lessons more seriously.

Emails and texts continued to flow back and forth between us; the internet was buzzing with an onslaught of constant, eager messages. I felt such a thrill every time I saw his name pop up in the corner of my computer screen. Maybe we were so interested in each other's worlds because we weren't an obvious match. Opposites attract, after all. But he was intelligent, good-looking, and charming. I fancied him, and he seemed to be genuinely interested in me, a much older man from England. Neither the 29-year age gap nor geographical difference seemed to worry him.

Then we discovered Skype where we could hear each other's voices and see faces at the same time. How quickly things changed for us with that invention. I was working at the theatre in Chichester most weekdays, but I was at home alone on Sundays, with my three cats. This turned out to be the best day for us to chat. It was purely thanks to the great generosity of his best friend, who owned an internet café and offered us several free calls. He preferred to chat at weekends because he could speak freely in English. He said it would look, and sound, odd to locals if they heard him speaking English in public at the café. On Sundays though there were usually not many people around to hear him chat. It was a perfect scenario.

Those Sunday internet calls were incredibly special. It made a world of difference to see his beautiful face up close, even if it was behind a screen. It was clear that we liked each other. I had let go of any expectations as soon as we first clicked. I wasn't naive – we lived thousands of miles apart, how likely was it that our chats would amount to anything? We were becoming pen pals. Nothing more was expected to happen. I was simply happy just to talk, for as long as it lasted. But then the days turned to weeks, and weeks turned to months, and feelings I hadn't felt in such a long time stirred within me, every time I spoke to this angelic man. Was it possible we were falling in love?

He was a Muslim, and I was a Christian. Not that we had deep conversations about either of our religions during our internet courtship – I guessed it was not the most immediate topic people on Gaydar usually asked each other about. But I knew that my faith was not as deeply rooted as his. Not that he spent too much time in the mosque during his teenage years, from what he told me.

His family called him Mo, short for Mohammed, and he had another Arabic name of Rassim, which I believe means architect, or planner. I told him, as a joke, that he had come down from heaven to meet me, so I referred to him as "my angel". How cheesy.

It was clear, after a few months, that being virtual pen pals was not enough for us. We wanted to meet each other face to face. But how the hell could this happen? He had no visa, or hope of obtaining one, to visit the UK.

Perhaps our internet love affair was simply a lost cause.

CHAPTER NINE

The season at Chichester Festival Theatre in 2005 was in repertoire, so I had a ten-day break coming up in August when I was not appearing in any shows. I had been planning to spend my time working on chores in my garden, the smelliest of which would involve clearing debris from the bottom of my huge pond. But when I realised my ten-day break from work would coincide with the 30th birthday of my new love interest, I knew my green-fingered endeavours would have to wait.

His upcoming birthday seemed to be a golden opportunity to arrange our first meeting. A test, in a way, to see if our online relationship was strong enough to flourish in real life. If it was not, then we would keep in touch as friends. There was nothing to lose and everything to gain.

I wondered if my friends and colleagues would understand my plan to meet this man after a six-month courtship made up of Skype calls, texts, and emails. I had never fully contemplated meeting another serious life partner after Robert died. Not yet, even if he had been dead for 13 years by now. What would he think about my intentions with this man if he were still around? Would he approve? His approval on various matters in my life, including a holiday with a new lover, did still matter.

"I have some time off in August," I announced during our next Sunday Skype session, pausing before I put forward my proposal. For a moment I felt nervous, knowing that what I was about to ask wasn't going to be easy to arrange. "How would you feel about me planning a little holiday, so we can meet?"
He gasped. "Do you really think that's a possibility?"
"I think it's a great idea, especially if we can include your 30th birthday when we're away," I said, relieved at his infectious enthusiasm.
"I'd love to be with you on my birthday," he said softly, grinning through the grainy webcam.

I very boldly suggested we meet in Paris. As he was a French-speaking person, it did seem to make perfect sense to meet up in the City of Light. Plus, I could easily hop on the Eurostar and be in my potential lover's arms in a matter of hours. As it happened, I still had the keys to my friends' apartment in Paris, where I often did cat-sitting duty for them when on their holidays. But for my young man, getting out of Algeria to visit anywhere in Europe was impossible without a Schengen visa. And trying to get holiday visas anywhere at short notice was not easy. So, Paris for a week was out of the question.

"If I can't get a Schengen visa to leave here, then maybe you can come to meet me in one of the North African countries," he suggested. "I can travel anywhere here with no restrictions." The perfect answer to our dilemma.

"Yes!" I said excitedly, "I never thought of North Africa at all. But where?" Algeria, as far as I knew, was not really a holiday destination for Brits.

"What about us meeting in Tunisia?" I suggested. "It's right next door to you." I knew Tunisia was a popular tourist destination – over the years I had seen piles of glossy holiday brochures showcasing pictures of white sand Tunisian beaches.

"I've never been, but I can get there," he said excitedly.

I researched online, searching for the right place for hours. I wanted a hotel next to those sugary sandy beaches I had seen in the brochures, and I found one called Tej Marhaba in the city of Sousse. It was a palace, right by the sea – perfect for a romantic holiday in what looked like paradise.

I only told a few of my friends exactly where I was going and who I was going there with. I didn't want anyone to rain on my plans to meet with this young man. Then again, I didn't actually care what people thought, anyway. I was going for it, regardless of their opinions.

Crystal-clear arrangements were made at both ends. I was flying from Gatwick, and he was going for a cheaper option by train. His plan was to travel from his hometown up north to Algiers, the capital, and from there he would take a train across the country to the border with Tunisia. Sounded simple enough to me.

The day arrived for our separate journeys to Sousse. My flight was at 11.00am, but I arrived at the airport early, well before 9.00am, of course. I'm always early. I texted him to see where he was on his journey, he replied to say he was already on board a train from Algiers to the Tunisian border. It was a long slog – more than 800 miles – and he was sweltering in close to 40-degree heat with no air conditioning. I felt hot just thinking about it. I had no idea how he coped with such an uncomfortable journey.

Meanwhile, I was in the comparative luxury of the Gatwick departure lounge. The usual pre-holiday jitters intensified by the thought of finally seeing this gorgeous, smiley man up close.

After wandering around the airport for a while, perusing duty-free and picking up a posh bottle of cologne for my new beau, my flight was called over the Tannoy. I gathered my bags and embarked on the trek along the seemingly endless walkway to my gate.

I hauled my suitcase along the final stretch of corridor just as the sign ahead of me began to flash green for boarding. That's when it happened. Seconds before I joined the queue of boarding passengers, I received the fateful message.

"I'm at the border with Algeria and Tunisia," I read, under my breath, "the guards are holding me. They think I am on a list of suspected persons. They are not letting me enter."
I stared at the little green screen of my Nokia, feeling a hot flash creep across my scalp, rereading the message several times before it sunk in.
"What the *fuck* is he telling me?" I exploded out loud. In times of stress, I use quite an array of swear words to help me through. This was no exception; all my favourites flew freely from my mouth.

Eager holiday-goers waiting to board their planes were rushing past me as I stood frozen to the spot, completely flustered. I was in some sort of hideous nightmare holiday scenario. My lovely, smiley, charming person, a criminal? Surely not.

Final calls for my flight were announced, but I still could not move. I was numb. I looked down at my feet, willing them to take a step forward. But my brand-new holiday trainers appeared to be glued to the floor.

"Sir? Are you boarding?" The flight attendant behind the desk looked at me quizzically, presumably concerned that I was having some sort of episode. I didn't blame her.

"Yes, sorry," I replied with a cough. My mouth was so dry I could barely swallow, whereas the crack of my arse was decidedly damp as I had begun to sweat with fear into my new designer underwear. At last regaining control of my legs, I traipsed up the stairs to the open plane door. A grinning young girl greeted me with, "Welcome aboard sir, enjoy your flight!" (Are you kidding me?)

What the hell did he mean by a suspected person? There had to be a simple explanation, surely. Perhaps it was a mistaken identity error; perhaps he was now on his way to the luxury hotel I had chosen for us. If so, considering I had a three-hour flight ahead of me, he could still arrive well before I would.

But whatever I told myself, I could not settle for the whole butt-clenching flight. The excitement and anticipation one normally feels when going on holiday with someone gorgeous for the first time was very much absent. I didn't eat a morsel of the soggy plane food because I felt so nauseous; I thought my head would explode at any minute trying to understand the mind-boggling situation I found myself facing.

I was still in an anxious state when we landed at Monastir Airport. As soon as I grabbed my luggage from the rickety carousel, I rushed through the arrivals hall and out the automatic front doors. The baking heat of the August sun only added to the sweat that now seemed to cover every inch of my body, but at least outside the terminal I finally had a few bars of signal on my phone. I started to text him frantically, but my attempts to make contact were futile. It had been hours since his last reply.

My mind was racing nineteen to the dozen. I had no idea what to do. I didn't know how to behave naturally as I carried my case towards the airport transfer shuttle bus which was waiting to take me to my hotel. I was, with huge difficulty, trying to appear as nonchalant as possible, but inside my head, I was screaming "SHIT, FUCK, BOLLOCKS," like a mantra.

Where was he? Who is he? No reply, no reply, no reply. Bollocks.

I felt like a total idiot for thinking the holiday would work out for me. What on earth would I tell everyone if I made it all the way to Tunisia and my man did not? It would be such a mortifying tale to relate to my friends at the theatre when I returned to work the following week.

I couldn't believe I had even tried dating again, after nine years with Robert. "You silly old sod," I said to myself, "what the hell are you doing here?!"

It was about 9.00pm, local time, and I felt like I was about to vomit on the bus ride to the posh hotel, although with no food in my stomach, it was hardly possible. I saw nothing of what may have been beautiful countryside outside, I just stared straight ahead in a daze. The only sensation I felt was the warm Tunisian evening air rushing over me through an open window. I was numb to everything else.

The bus arrived at the hotel in Sousse, which looked even more impressive than the pictures. In the foyer, there were huge, lit floral displays cascading down from colossal marble pillars, and the reception desk was nestled under enormous shrubbery that shaded the seating areas. I was used to staying in Premier

Inns in the UK, so it was a rather grand place by comparison. A perfect location indeed for a romantic first meeting. But my companion was nowhere to be seen.

I handed my passport over to the gentleman at the tree-lined reception desk. "Has my friend arrived yet?" I asked nervously. I was physically and emotionally exhausted, but I tried to appear as polite and friendly as possible. The tall, sour-faced reception clerk, however, did not make the same effort.
"No sir, no one else here, no news," he said curtly.
"Well, I expect he will be arriving very soon, we were on different flights..." I began to explain, but the disinterested receptionist barely lifted his eyes from his computer screen as his fingers clacked along the keyboard, so I gave up. We weren't off to a good start. I signed the register; he handed me the keys and said flatly, as though bored by my presence: "Take the lift to the room on the eighth floor, sir".

I continued to text my absent companion as I left the lobby. I half expected him to leap out from behind one of the giant pillars in the foyer and reveal that it had all been some sort of ill-thought-out joke. But no, there was still no sign of him, and no messages either. It was dawning on me that I might truly be on this holiday alone.

I found the main lift to my floor and the doors opened to reveal hideously unforgiving, mirror-clad walls. "Jesus Christ, you look bloody *awful*," I said to my reflection, in total shock at the haggard, grey, English guy staring back at me. Looking like a forlorn deer in incredibly unflattering headlights.

I let out a pitiful sigh, pressed the buttons to the eighth floor, and dragged my luggage, and my feet, from the lift to the suite. I felt desperately alone.

At least my room was superb, and bigger than I expected. There were two huge beds, each flanked by enormous bedside lamps on either side. There was a balcony beyond floor-to-ceiling sliding glass doors, so I ventured outside to find a spectacularly large seating area with a view overlooking the manicured gardens below and pathways down to the sea. The night breeze carried the wonderful, sweet smells of jasmine flowers. It should have been a serene moment. It wasn't.

"Where in God's name is he?" I growled at the empty night around me. Then I had an awful thought that he could be sitting in a dark, sweaty prison cell somewhere at that very moment, which sent my stomach into a cartwheel. I watched my textless phone that I had left charging on the desk in the bedroom as I paced around, expecting it to ring any second.

While I waited for news, in my typically tidy way, I wasted no time unpacking my clothes and hanging them in the spacious closet. The rational side of my brain had forced me to accept that I must stay there for a week, even if he never arrived. So, I placed my toiletries in the bathroom, which really was a splendid room. There were beautifully stylish marble fittings everywhere, with white, soft, fluffy towels neatly folded beside the sink. Oh my. Even in this time of great stress, I was able to fawn over a truly sumptuous bathroom. I must be gay.

I had no idea what to do with myself. I was sure I was wearing the carpet out, walking about so much. Although it was extremely late at night in England, I decided to ring my dearest friend and theatre agent, Lesley. She was in the loop, weeks before, regarding my intentions to come to Tunisia and holiday with this guy.

"It's a good plan, go and have some fun in a sunny climate with someone handsome," she had urged, "you've got nothing to lose". She was always very supportive and had seen me through the difficult months of nursing Robert, so she was happy I was engaging in a new romance all these years later. She understood that this trip was a rather daring thing for me to be undertaking, compared to my usually cautious approach to life.

"I feel like such an idiot," I confessed to Lesley on the other end of the line after I had explained what had happened. I didn't mention the suspected person fiasco. That side of things was too much to have explained over the phone, and she might have freaked out. I know I must have sounded rather odd mumbling about my confusion and disappointment. But I needed to vent. I was still baffled as to what was happening and I had no clue what I should do next.

Once I had finished my anxious rambling, Lesley said: "Look, sweetheart, it might help you to rest and see how things pan out in the morning. You sound tired, you need a bit of sleep." I thanked her and hung up.

It was coming up to midnight and I was going out of my mind. I flopped on to one of the vast, luxurious beds, although, as exhausted as I was, I knew that sleep was not yet on the cards – how could it be? Fully conscious, I stared at the off-white ceiling until my eyes went out of focus. I tossed and turned in my anxious state, trying, and failing, to calm down enough to drift off. I felt like I was appearing in the middle of a scene from a hideous horror movie, desperately waiting for the director to yell *"CUT!"*

CHAPTER TEN

The shrill ring of the bedside telephone made me leap out of my skin. I fumbled in the dark to grab the old-fashioned receiver, turning on the enormous bedside lamp as I answered on the third ring. It was the snotty receptionist with his suspicious, superior manner, calling to inform me that there was someone who wished to speak to me.

I took a deep breath and braced myself for the news that I had been dreading: my young man was calling from prison and needed help getting out.

"Hello?" I said tentatively, nervously fidgeting with the telephone cord in my left hand. Then I sat up with such speed that I gave myself a head rush. It was him. But he wasn't calling from some distant holding cell, he was calling from the phone in the lobby. I couldn't believe my ears. The man I had travelled such a distance to meet was downstairs in the hotel foyer.

I was completely flustered at his sudden arrival. I ran to the wardrobe in a tizzy to swiftly change into something more alluring while he made his way up to the eighth floor. I didn't want to wear pyjamas for our first meeting.

There was a knock on the door. My heart thumped against my ribs. I opened the door, and there standing in the hallway in front of me, was my smiling angel.

"Finally, you're here!" I said with a nervous laugh.

"Oh, I am so very sorry it has taken so long for me to get here," he replied with a sigh. I could tell that he was trying to gauge my mood. Before the phone rang, I had been close to tearing my hair out, it's true. But at that moment, as he stood in front of me, I felt utterly content.

"Don't worry," I said, holding out my arms to him, "you're here now".

We hugged for an eternity, laughing as we held each other tight to relieve the tension of the last few hours. It was such a relief to finally be together, in the same room, at long last.

He dumped his suitcase in the hallway, looked around the room briefly and said: "This is nice, but I'm desperate to smoke, let's go on this huge balcony for a cigarette". We stepped outside, lit cigarettes, and found an ashtray, and I asked him what on earth had happened on the journey.

"My original plan was okay," he began, pausing to take a draw of his cigarette before he continued: "I took a flight from Oran, it's the nearest airport from my home, to take me to Algiers". He leant over the balcony for a moment, distracted by the sweet, musky smell of jasmine that filled the air. "We have this same jasmine flower at home too, it's lovely," he said.

I inhaled the flowery perfume with him and felt myself finally begin to relax. "So, tell me more," I said reaching out to hold his left hand as he smoked with his right.

"Well, the train started in Algiers, and it's a very old train and a *very* long journey. My God, I was so hot and there were many smelly people on it, too." He scrunched his nose in disapproval.

"That sounds dreadful," I said, "I was going through agonies at Gatwick after reading your text before I got on my plane".

"Oh! That message, I know, I am so sorry," he said sincerely. I smiled and stroked his arm in acceptance of his apology. The horrors of that day now felt like a distant memory.

"Anyway," he said with an air of excitement, "let me tell you everything". I settled in for the story.

"The actual train never goes right into the city of Tunis at all but stops about 30 kilometres from the passport area."

"Why does that happen?" I asked.

He waved his cigarette hand and rolled his eyes in exaggerated exasperation. "Ugh, it's so ancient a system, it's not sophisticated at all," he explained. "The passengers get off the train and pile into minicabs that drive everyone the last few miles to the passport check station."

He puffed on his cigarette as he continued his story. "There the people queue up to get passports stamped, then get back into the same cabs and drive into the capital. We pay for the full journey before we get in."

I tried to visualise the events as he described them. The whole ordeal sounded like a complete pain in the arse already.

"I had everything ready when we lined up at the passport control booth," he said, "then someone looked at my passport and asked me if I could show papers to prove that my dad's name was the same family name as my passport."

"That's a weird thing to ask, surely."

"Those guys are stupid, unintelligent idiots!" he fumed. "Why ask a question like that? I told them, I can contact my dad and he can fax them anything they need. It was all total bullshit, of course, I realise now, but I tried to be polite." He stubbed out his cigarette. "Can we go downstairs and get some drinks somewhere? I'm so thirsty."

"Sure, we can," I said, "let's go out".

The holiday jitters were back. I couldn't wait to begin our adventure together. We called the lift to the ground floor and stepped out into the beautiful gardens. It was well past midnight, but the air was comfortably warm. We found a quiet bar on the hotel grounds and ordered drinks and a few nibbles to go with them.

"Tell me more please, I want the whole story," I said, relaxed enough to indulge in the drama a little.

He took a huge glug from an icy glass of coke, as soon as the waiter set it on the table in front of him and relaxed into his chair. "Well, they placed me to one side from the other passengers at the passport area and said they wanted to check my name against lists they have to see if I was on a terror suspect list."

My mouth fell open in disbelief. "Oh! Hell no," I said, "did you say anything else to them then?"

"No, I didn't. I was so bloody shocked and a bit scared, so I stood to one side in silence."

We soon were well-established in the quiet bar, and completely comfortable with each other. Our holiday had gotten off to a rocky start, but, if anything, the hideous ordeal negated any chance of awkward silences or lulls in conversation. I wanted to put my arms around him and give him a hug, but I held back in case someone saw us. I felt I had to be careful. I knew that physical contact in public would be frowned upon – or worse – so we didn't touch each other at all. I knew homosexuality was criminalised in many Islamic countries, like Tunisia, so I wasn't going to rock the boat by trying to hold his hand. I didn't want to do anything to ruin our first holiday together. Besides, sitting so close together for the first time, after months of seeing him behind a screen, was rather special anyway.

"They ignored me standing alone away from the other passengers for ages. I did not know what I was supposed to do," he said solemnly, continuing his saga.

"I wish I had known all this was happening to you," I replied with concern.

"The thing was, I couldn't call you or text you because I had run out of credit." By now he was smoking furiously again, in between slurps of coca cola, as he continued his tale. "It was so awful not being able to call you and tell you about my delay. I'm sorry."

"Please, you don't have to apologise to me," I said, leaning in closer. This whole ordeal must have been incredibly upsetting for him. "So, what happened next?"

"Well, people were staring at me standing alone and I honestly wanted to cry, then an older couple talked to me because they saw I was upset. They suggested I might give the guards a bit of money to see if they would stamp my passport and let me go."

"So, what did you do?"

"That's when I saw the minicab I already paid for drive off full of passengers, leaving me behind. I was so angry, I just wanted out of there, so I took the advice of the nice couple and opened my wallet when I saw a guard looking over at me."

"They were only after a bribe then?"

"Obviously they were, I could see the guards were watching me doing this, then, just seconds later, they came forward and had my passport already stamped and let me go through."

"What, it was that easy?" I spluttered.

"Yes, yes it was that easy. It must happen often," he said with a shrug.

Bastard border guards, "Welcome to Tunisia", I don't think. What a completely awful experience he endured simply to meet me. He deserved a medal.

After six months of talking online, and a harrowing, arduous journey, we were now taking a romantic stroll through stunning gardens by the North African coast in the moonlight. Who'd have thought it?

We talked and walked for a little while, smoked some strange foreign cigarettes, and eventually returned to the room on the eighth floor to sleep together for the first time. Having known each other for several months by this stage, it felt completely natural, being together in that way. We were not strangers to each other; there were no awkward moments.

Not many couples face such a start to their relationship; not many couples face such an ending.

CHAPTER ELEVEN

The next morning, after the rollercoaster of a day before, we were both ravenous, unsurprisingly. We entered the large hotel dining area for our first meal together, and there facing us was a sumptuous – expansive – breakfast buffet. We couldn't wait to dive in.

"Let's sit in that corner away from the others," he said. We filled our plates with all sorts of food and ate well, but each time we saw a different staff member, we knew they were scrutinising us. You could tell they were thinking, "Why is this older English tourist sitting with a much younger, local man?" We must have appeared as an odd couple to some. Perhaps they were thinking that I had a paid holiday companion with me.

But after a few days, the staff seemed to realise we were together for an entire week's holiday. Not just a one-night stand. Thankfully the odd looks disappeared, and I began to feel less uncomfortable. Except, of course, whenever I saw the snotty receptionist, who gave us a daily disapproving look as we collected our room keys.

My holidays were always in Europe, so everything about this trip was quite a different experience for me. As my man spoke French and Arabic fluently, he was able to explain anything that I was unfamiliar with. He explained shops, and street signs, and knew directions to various places we could visit, such as the souk in the centre of town. I had never visited such a place in my life. He pointed out the mouth-watering aromas of endless spices from different stalls that were put out for sale in huge pots. The smells of cooking coming from the surrounding local restaurants and street food sellers were tantalising, too.

When we passed a shop that looked like a cross between a delicatessen and a butcher, he pointed at some meat in the window and said: "Can we buy some? I want to taste it". I was surprised he was so interested – it just looked like regular sliced ham to me. Not quite the packet stuff we buy from Sainsbury's, but similar.

"Yes, I'll get some for us, are you coming inside too?"

He declined to enter the shop with me, so I went in alone. It never occurred to me that this meat was a pork product and therefore haram, forbidden in the Islamic faith, which is why he shied away from buying it with me.

I knew from my Jewish friends that pig products were forbidden in their faith. Although many of my Jewish mates, I have to say, do love a bacon sarnie. But at the time, I knew next to nothing about my lover's religion. It never occurred to me that it was forbidden in Islam too. I only started to understand the meaning of haram a lot later in the relationship.

We were on a romantic getaway, simply enjoying each other's company for the first time. We didn't delve into each other's faiths; we never talked about what wasn't permitted in his religion or mine. I am sure there were many topics we could have discussed, including homosexuality – also forbidden – but we did not.

In the streets of Sousse, I saw local people looking quizzically at us, even European tourists did, too. This worried me a little when we were strolling in areas further away from the hotel, although my lover didn't appear to be concerned in the slightest. That day we had wandered quite a distance from the main tourist areas, and it was swelteringly hot, so I was in need of a cooling refreshment when I spotted a little parlour that made its own ice cream.

"Look at that place," I said, my mouth beginning to water just looking at the soft pastel-coloured peaks on display, "let me buy you one".

My love flashed his trademark smile before asking politely for his favourite flavour. We each took a seat on the terrace outside the store, racing to eat the deliciously fresh scoops before they turned to puddles in the sun.

All of a sudden, I was aware of young eyes looking at us. There were crowds of kids hanging around in the street by this parlour. It appeared we were a kind of novelty tourist attraction to them. They were giggling and talking about us – I didn't need to speak the language to know that.

"Why are they so interested in watching us eating ice cream?" I asked, a little self-consciously. My smiley man didn't say anything, offering a simple shrug as he continued eating. He didn't seem to be affected by the kids' attention, as far as I could tell at least. But this strange, uncomfortable feeling stayed with me for a long time. The whole scenario reminded me of a scene from a Tennessee Williams play, *Suddenly Last Summer*.

After a morning of exploring, we couldn't wait to lounge on the beach – it was too hot to wander the city after lunch. It was a short walk through the hotel grounds, carrying towels, cigarettes, a lighter, plus a refreshing drink or two, past the massive indoor swimming pool and down to the sugary beach which was dotted with coloured umbrellas.

"I have never walked on sand like this in my life," I said with great delight. It was so unlike the pebbles that I was used to seeing on the south coast of England.

"This is very similar to the beaches in Oran, where I swam with my friends at university," he said, smiling. "Some days we stayed in the sea for hours, talking and jumping up and down fighting each other."

"You must be a great swimmer then," I said.

"No, I'm hopeless," he replied with a laugh, "I just like being in the water".

For us, lying on sunbeds under hotel canopies on the soft white sand was one of our favourite parts of each day. We smoked like a pair of chimneys, and we never ran out of things to talk about. It was utter bliss. I addressed him as Angel during these moments in the sun. It seemed a perfectly natural name to use at intimate times together.

We picked a different brand of Tunisian cigarettes to smoke every day – there was quite an array to choose from. The unusual smell from any local cigarette always encapsulates a distinct feeling of whatever country you are in. Most of them were okay, but one brand, in particular, tasted like camel dung. He laughed a lot when I told him that.

In the evenings, after dinner in our hotel, we'd smoke that day's cigarettes and drink coffee on lounge chairs in the orangery underneath ginormous palm trees. I had presumed that Tunisian coffee would be amazing, especially in this grand hotel. Sadly, the Tej Marhaba's supply was awful. But we didn't care – the setting and the company made for an enjoyable evening, regardless. The hotel, always beautifully lit at night, turned into a fairy-tale palace. I felt as if I was on a film set with my smiley person beside me. It was so wonderfully surreal.

One day, we were having our usual stewed coffee in the orangery when my love spotted a young local boy selling trinkets near the doors to the gardens. He walked over, and, curiously, had quite a long conversation with the boy before he returned to our table.

"Here, this is for you," he said with a shy smile. It was a little silver wristband. He had asked the boy to scrape – rather crudely – my first name on the widest part of the band.

"Thank you, you didn't have to do that," I said, turning it over in my palm. I've kept hold of it all these years, even though it's a cheap, tacky thing. I treasure it mostly because there was little cash left in his wallet for a gift for me, seeing as he had already handed much of his money over to the crooked border guards for his release. It was such a kind, thoughtful gesture.

CHAPTER TWELVE

Our third day in Tunisia was marked to meet up with Paul Van Der Wheele, one of my oldest friends and former housemate, from Brighton. Paul was retired by now, but back in Brighton, a few months before, we met up for a drink and gossip in his pretty little cottage near the station.

"I've been offered a movie again as production accountant," he announced, gleefully.

"What?" I said, "I thought you'd already gone into retirement last year, you said you'd had enough."

"Well, yes," he said, "I did, and as I've worked on so many films over the years, I thought it was time to put my feet up."

"Yes, you've certainly done that," I agreed. "But honestly, Paul, I know you've been missing that sort of life, haven't you?"

"You know me," he said, "I have been mulling it over, and the money would be very good," he chuckled. "So, yes, I'm seriously thinking about the offer."

"Good for you. Are the locations all over the place as usual?"

"Well luckily for me it's in the one place for several months, in a town called Hammamet."

"Where's that? I've never heard of it."

"I'm not that sure exactly, but it's somewhere in Tunisia."

I gawped at him for a moment, then screamed: "You've got to be kidding me!"

Poor Paul jumped out of his skin.

"Dear, Tunisia is where I'm going to meet that guy I told you about."

"No way," he said, shocked, "have you arranged that already?"

I told him that I had booked a hotel in an area called Sousse, and suggested we look it up on his atlas. We checked the map excitedly and compared dates in our diaries, and we were both completely gobsmacked as they synchronised perfectly. What an amazing, surprising piece of news for us both.

Paul was much more adventurous than I was, so he constantly encouraged me to go ahead with plans to meet someone new after Robert died. Although, even so, I'm sure he could hardly believe I was flying halfway across the world to meet a man. He was great friends with Robert; he adored him. But he was a good friend to me and wished so much for me to move on with my life and be happy.

I was so thrilled about the possibility that someone I knew so well would be meeting my handsome Algerian. Was this a coincidence that both of us were planning to be in Tunisia at the time? No, I say it often, I do not believe in them.

Soon after I arrived in Sousse, I called Paul in Hammamet to arrange a meeting at his place, a boutique hotel on the beach there called The Sinbad. When the meeting day arrived, I was nervous about one of my oldest, closest friends meeting my young man. Would he think we were suited, or an odd match? Paul never held back on his opinion on anything, particularly when it concerned his friends taking a new partner, so I knew, at some point, he was going to tell me exactly what he thought.

It was a short taxi drive to The Sinbad and when we arrived it was clear I needn't have worried – Paul realised that my new man was nervous about meeting him, my long-term friend, for the very first time, so he was especially pleasant and welcoming. It was such a relief watching them shake hands, grinning at each other. It really was such a milestone event for me.

"I really want to take you both out to lunch," Paul said to us as we sipped on coffee in his hotel (which was miles better than the bitter gloop served at ours). "There's this great little place called Da Franco's. The food is fab, you'll love it. And I'm earning shitloads of money at the moment – let's go and spend it." He flashed a cheeky grin. It was such a thrill to see him including my guy into our circle.

So, after coffee, we took a taxi to the restaurant, which was in a beautiful, secluded courtyard, decorated with olive trees that cast dappled shade over all the tables. It was a stunning location – a very exclusive place by my standards.

"Shall I order my favourite wine with lunch?" Paul asked.

Still ignorant of the idea of haram, I was totally unaware of the restrictions on the consumption of alcohol for Muslims. My young man never indicated any taboo, so the three of us got stuck into a crisp bottle of white while practically drooling over tempura vegetables and calamari – an amazing dish at the best of times, but this was very fine-dining squid. Paul talked the entire time, telling jokes, making us laugh with silly tales of filming days, which my man was really interested to hear about.

This first meeting was a huge success, but I do remember thinking at the time just how unusual it was, that my oldest mate and I were having a meal together, with this person I met on the internet in a faraway country. It was an unusual scenario by my usual standard of living. Was this a good omen for our future together? It had to be.

CHAPTER THIRTEEN

The holiday was already off to a spectacular start – in my wildest dreams, I couldn't have imagined better – but I wanted to do something particularly special for my love's 30th birthday. After all, neither of us knew if, or when, we would celebrate another together.

"What do you think of having dinner away from the hotel?" I asked, on the morning of his birthday, as we wandered around an area of fancy restaurants in Sousse. He beamed in response.

"I'd quite like to try this one," he said eagerly as we passed a charming little place by the sea. All the tables were outside, and it looked exclusive but not out of my pocket. So that evening, we chose a quiet spot by the water's edge.

"Shall I order champagne with our meal?" I asked with a grin. Although I'm not a big drinker, I wanted to make the evening special.

His eyes lit up. "Yes please," he said, "I've never tasted it before."

I ordered a bottle of bubbly to impress him. This was much to the delight of the waiter (I guessed he was on commission).

My excitement was short-lived, as what arrived inside a large ice bucket was not delicious French fizz but an inferior bottle of Asti Spumante. I'll admit I have little knowledge of most alcoholic beverages, but even I knew that what arrived at our table was most definitely not champagne.

There was a big smile and lots of head nodding from the waiter as he presented it to us, as if it was nectar from the heavens. I didn't have the heart to complain or ask for him to replace it. I certainly did not want to make a fuss in front of my man. Instead, in a terribly British manner, I smiled and accepted the bottle, and nodded back to the beaming waiter. To be honest, the taste did not matter – it could have been filled with seawater as far as I was concerned. All that mattered was that we were spending this time together.

Two nights later, our final evening together was spent walking around the jasmine gardens, smoking and chatting, a nightly routine we'd come to treasure. I'd been trying to imagine what to say to him about our future once our week was over. We'd built such a deep connection over a relatively short period on the internet, and now, after meeting face to face, neither of us wanted our time together to end. But what could we say, what could we do? It was a given that we had no intention of ending this with a "goodbye it's been nice, see you around" sort of farewell.

When the next morning arrived to end our first holiday together, we had our last shitty coffee and a cigarette in the lounge. He collected his bags from the foyer, and we waited for his taxi ride to the airport. I was taking a much later flight the same day, so I was going to stay on in the hotel for a few more hours.

Earlier in the week, thoughts of the return journey my lover would have to take back to Algeria, alone, haunted me. I couldn't let him go home by train. I didn't want him to have a similarly traumatic episode with the border guards after having such a splendid holiday together. So, I bought an airline ticket back to Oran (his university city) on the Mediterranean coast. Then there was just a drive to his home. It was his birthday present. I told him it was the best I could do to soften the blow of the incident with the corrupt guards. If he was safely on a plane, it would put my mind at rest. Surprisingly, the price of the plane ticket was amazingly cheap, considering it would fly him close to 1,000 miles. I couldn't get a train ticket from Brighton to Manchester for that sort of price.

It was impossible for either of us to know what to say during those final few minutes together. He was tearful when the taxi arrived in the hotel driveway. I too felt rather weepy, but my very English stiff upper lip held me back. This had been an amazingly successful first meeting, but now we were saying goodbye not knowing what the future held for us.

He lifted his belongings into the taxi, and we hugged each other one last time. As his taxi drove away to the airport I saw my man, sitting in the back seat, turn around to look at me through the rear window, waving and crying, his radiant smile replaced by a quivering pout. It was the classic, film-worthy shot: a weeping person being driven away unwillingly from a loved one. And I knew I did truly love him in that moment. It was almost too much for me to bear. As he faded out of sight, my own tears began to flow.

I stayed in the hotel, wandering around the grounds thinking about the past few days with him. Mostly wondering what the future could hold for us now. I was decidedly low of spirit. I drank yet another cup of shitty hotel coffee and smoked the last of the local cigarettes he left behind with me. I didn't throw away the empty packet. I have it with me now, Cristal brand, a Tunisian keepsake.

This is not the end; I kept telling myself. There must be much more to come.

CHAPTER FOURTEEN

Flying home to Gatwick alone was dreadful. I was haunted by thoughts of the future: was our relationship destined to be a holiday romance, nothing more? The past week confirmed that we wanted to be together, but the odds were very much against us, and there were thousands of miles between us.

As soon as I settled back at home, I had to return for the last few performances at Chichester Theatre. I was excited to get back; the theatre has always felt like a second home to me. I barely made it through the door of the green room before I was bombarded with questions about my new beau from nosey actor mates.

I had told a select few about my holiday, and a little bit about the man I was meeting, but to some, he was a total unknown, a stranger, and so arranging to meet him seemed a dodgy plan in the first place.
"Why would you, of all people, do such a thing, travelling so far to meet this guy?" someone asked me.
My holiday liaison, to my theatre pals, seemed to be very out of keeping with the person they thought they knew. I could see their point of view – I wouldn't venture to a club to meet a man, but, somehow, I would venture all the way to Africa?

It didn't take long for the line of inquiry to become more invasive.
"Did you have 'fun' together darling?" one friend asked, with a wink.
This, of course, was their way of asking if there was anything sexual going on between us. I was discreet with my replies to such questions – it was none of their business, as far as I was concerned. Besides, a gentleman doesn't kiss and tell.

"Well, what does he look like?" asked another.

I produced some holiday photographs. All clothed pictures – to their dismay, I'm sure – of us exploring the sights. But they seemed to approve, nonetheless.

"Yes, he's a dish all right," one girl said.

Then one friend asked the most basic of questions which stopped me in my tracks: "What's his name?"

For months I had referred to him almost exclusively as 'my Angel'. I thought it sweet, but it was far too personal, and cheesy to outsiders, to share. So, without really thinking about it, I simply said: "His name is Angelo". The name came out quite easily – I just, rather crudely, stuck an 'o' on the end of 'Angel'. But it was accepted by the group, especially as, as they could see from the photographs, he was an Italian-looking dish.

The final question, the one that stuck with me, long after our rehearsals were finished, was the most obvious: "Will it last, dear?" Perhaps I should have said to them: "Oh! It was only a holiday romance, you know. We're not keeping in touch." That would have been one way to stop the onslaught of questions.

Of course, there was not a single idea in my head as to how I could continue the relationship. I hadn't thought of the bigger picture – after all, I'd only just left him in Tunisia three days before.

That evening, I phoned Angelo – who chuckled when I told him I had referred to him as such, and gladly adopted the name – to discuss the best plan of action for him to come to the UK. He needed to secure a visa, that much we were sure of, but we had no idea where to begin. Neither of us had applied for any kind of visa before. It turned out that the type of visa that could be applied for was dictated by the country you were coming from. We both imagined a holiday visa to England would be the best option, assuming that once here on holiday, he could apply for an extension to stay on. How totally naive we both were to think that scenario would work out. It was a rotten, ill-thought-out idea.

He called me to say he had found an application. The Spanish inquisition-inspired form gave my inquisitive theatre mates a run for their money.

"I'll email it, so you can read the questions," he said. Filling in this expansive form was a daunting prospect – a dyslexic person's idea of hell. I could barely make sense of it.

"Some of these questions are so *stupid*," he complained.

"I know, but we have to be very careful about the answers," I said earnestly, "there can be no slip-ups".

I scrolled through the pages on my PC.

Why do you want to visit the UK?
What is the duration of your stay in the UK?
Who is covering your expenses?
Have you been to the UK before?
Do you intend to work in the UK?
Do you have relatives/friends in the UK?
What do you do?
Will you be travelling alone or with a group or family?
Where will you be staying in the UK?

I presumed as he would be staying with me, a respectable homeowner and older gentleman, at my address, it would surely cement a successful application.

Then there were questions relating to me, asking for details about the nature of our relationship, whether I was a family friend, and how exactly we came to be acquainted. Thinking it would help our case, I wrote something totally idiotic and completely untrue – I claimed I knew both his parents. But we had no intention of saying anything that would vaguely hint at a gay relationship. We both thought that doing so would halt any chances of success, especially considering the laws of the country he was applying from. We avoided saying that we met on a gay dating site and subsequently spent a holiday together.

Then came another spanner in the works.

"I've got to hand in the application myself," Angelo said dolefully, "I can't mail it. I've got to go to the nearest British Consulate."

A faff, I thought. But it got worse.

"There isn't one in Algeria, at all," he continued, "there appears to be only one British Consulate in the whole of North Africa, and it's in Tunis".

I couldn't believe my ears; I dreaded the thought of him making the same, perilous journey as he had just weeks before. It was a mammoth expedition, but he was eager to do it just so we could possibly be together again in England.

After a long slog from Algeria and an overnight in a cheap hotel in Tunis, the moment arrived. I called him just as he was about to enter the British Consulate grounds, clutching his application form tightly, along with his passport papers and photographs of the two of us on holiday, taken just a few weeks before.

"Wish me luck!" He was full of enthusiasm; I was a bag of nerves.

"Good luck, my love," I said, "call me as soon as you can".

They called him into a booth where he was scrutinised by a Consulate official who asked even more questions. Then he spent several hours in a lifeless waiting room while his fate was decided for him. He didn't even try to phone me. In the meantime, I was chewing on my nails back in Saltdean.

Then the moment arrived when he phoned me to give me the result. He didn't have to say much – I knew immediately from his voice that the news wasn't good.

"I am so very sorry," I said, feeling a lump rise in my throat. I was desperately upset, and I couldn't think of what to say to make him feel better. If he were a short journey away from me, I would have been there, to console and comfort him, and discuss our future possibilities. But we were oceans apart. It was a huge blow not getting the visa, but worse was not being at his side. That was unbearable.

"I was so upset, thinking that I may never be able to come to England," he told me on his homeward journey, "I thought my dream had ended". I felt as sick as a parrot hearing his gloomy thoughts.

Angelo and I talked endlessly over the next few days about what we could do next. It was so disheartening to be back at square one. I had no clue where to look, but we weren't giving up hope, even if the odds were against us. There had to be a way forward. Surely, someone we knew would have an idea or a plan of action – there had to be a solution somewhere.

One Saturday night, I was feeling particularly glum and emotionally drained, so I decided to ring one of my oldest pals, Elizabeth Edmiston, a wonderful actress and an even better friend. She was always up for a chat, even so late at night. Lizzie suffered from diabetes, which meant she was often ill and in bed with various physical ailments. But she was always a tonic to chat with when she was at home. I had witnessed her laugh and joke her way through several of her own near-death experiences. And when I visited her in the hospital over the years, she was always ready to give a comic performance for anyone watching.

Before my first visit to Tunisia, when Lizzie happened to be particularly poorly, I told her all about my plan to meet Angelo.
"You go for it, girl; you never know what it will lead to," she had said. Forever the optimist, even in her darkest days.

I first met Lizzie during my West End debut. The show was the first revival of Sandy Wilson's *The Boyfriend*, which was originally seen in London in 1954. I was over the moon to have landed my first big West End job, but I was also incredibly nervous as there was a fair amount of dancing in the show and I was not a dancer, to put it mildly. Lizzie knew this. She could see I was struggling to pick up the steps in the early rehearsals – I must have looked completely bewildered.

As a former ballerina, kind and talented Lizzie took me to one side and coached me herself so that I was able to master all the basic dance moves before we opened in London. She was there for me when I needed her and had been ever since.

At one point, Lizzie was living in Wandsworth with her then-boyfriend. I had a flat in the same house and we saw each other daily as my living room was directly above hers. As we were living in such close proximity for months, we knew most everything about each other's lives that was of any interest, be it private or professional. During our Wandsworth days, I cemented a great friendship with her. And I also experienced some of her awful cooking.

That Saturday night, I dialled her number, and she picked up immediately, as usual, as she was in bed watching the TV, with the phone at hand.
"Hello, Mavis, how are you?"
Lizzie was perhaps the campest lady I'd ever known. She gave female names to most of her male friends, and mine was Mavis – no idea why. She even referred to her husband, a lovely actor named Eric Carte, as Erica. She called him the name publicly and he, along with all her friends, seemed to have adopted it.

She was a warm, loving person; she had a heart of gold and was as funny as can be, on stage, and off. She told me some terrible jokes, then hurled endless abuse at me about my sad empty life living on the south coast alone while I laughed and shrieked at her stories. Then, when I was able to get a word in edgeways, I told her my tale of woe. She listened intently as I relayed our successful holiday together, how we wanted to continue to be together, the nightmare of the unsuccessful visa application to bring him to England, and how the distance between us seemed insurmountable.

"So, my dear, what the hell can we do? Where on earth can I find any help?" I asked, making no effort to hide the desperation in my voice. I realised it was decidedly dreary of me to offload my problems on to her so late in the evening. But she continued to listen.

After a while, once she'd thought over my plea for help, she said rather seriously:

"Well dear, I think I will make a call on Sunday morning and speak to May, to see if I can get any answers for you".

"May? Who the hell is May?" I asked her. I thought I knew all her girlfriends.

"Oh darling, I always call him May, you know me," she said. "He's my gay actor friend, Michael Cashman, you know who he is surely, darling?"

"Really Lizzie? I didn't know he was your mate," I said, rather shocked.

"Well dear," she continued, "now she's a European MP and supports many gay issues here and even international ones too. Maybe 'she' might know what you chaps can do for the best."

Lizzie spoke in such a matter-of-fact way, like an agony aunt giving advice. It was as if she solved these sorts of problems daily. It was also no surprise, given her fondness for feminine nicknames, that she addressed Michael Cashman as 'May'. Of course, I knew exactly who this man was – he once played the first openly gay character on Eastenders. So, I knew of his support for issues that faced the gay community. I was gobsmacked that she thought it was entirely acceptable to ring him at the weekend and ask him to help me, a total stranger. I assumed he would be rather busy with the European Parliament.

I was buzzing with excitement after talking with Lizzie this late evening. She completely lifted my spirits. I thanked her profusely, and we exchanged more jokes, quips, and insults before we said our goodbyes. Tired, but grinning like a Cheshire cat, I retired to bed more relaxed than I had been in weeks.

The next evening, after Sunday dinner, I had just settled down to watch some television when the landline phone rang.

"Hello, Trevor, I'm Michael Cashman. Lizzie tells me you have a problem. Do you want to tell me what the problem is?"

I was numb for a second and nearly dropped the phone. This was like my own Cinderella moment when the sweet fairy godmother appeared out of nowhere to come to my aid, only this time she was in the guise of Michael Cashman.

My mouth was sandpaper dry; I was completely tongue-tied. I tried to pull myself together, but I'm sure I sounded befuddled and a bit simple-minded. This was such a surprise. I had spoken to Lizzie less than 24 hours ago. I wasn't expecting him to get in touch so soon, if at all.

"Oh, hello Michael," I said timidly (perhaps I should have addressed him as May). "I wasn't too sure if Lizzie would contact you – thank you so much for calling me."

I relayed the entire story of my relationship with Angelo as succinctly as I could in my nervous state. Michael listened intently as I did so. Then came the verdict:

"I think you need to meet my mate, Barry O'Leary. He's an immigration lawyer based in Waterloo."

I could not believe my luck in talking to this man in the first place, now here he was, providing a possible solution to what I feared was an unsolvable problem. I was practically speechless, so our conversation was relatively short-lived, but Michael gave me an address and a phone number for Barry.

"Contact him ASAP, and go from there," he said kindly.

I thanked him profusely for his help and interest in our case, and hung up, with the phone shaking in my hand. A beaming smile split my face in two. God, how I wanted to give that man a big hug. He was fast becoming Saint Cashman in my eyes, perhaps I should light a candle in his name.

Dear, darling Lizzie, thank you.

CHAPTER FIFTEEN

I searched the internet for Barry, the solicitor in Waterloo, to find out more information about the sort of cases he dealt with. I learned that the firm had been involved with numerous global gay rights cases, some concerning the abuse, torture, and even death of LGBTQ+ people around the world. I worried if he would have any interest in our comparatively simple case.

I made an extremely panicky phone call to his office, laying out the bare facts of our situation once more. He said there was no guarantee he could help until he saw the bigger picture, but I think he could hear the anxiety in my voice, so he agreed to meet me at his firm's offices in Waterloo, just for a chat.

I was debilitatingly nervous on the walk from Waterloo station to the office to meet this man, so much so that when passing by the local street market stalls, I was physically sick behind an unsuspecting street vendor's vegetable display.

I've been interviewed by many of the industry's top theatre and television directors in my career. I've stood on stages performing to hundreds if not thousands of people, and all these things I have taken in my stride. So why was I so terrified to meet this solicitor man? I suppose I was scared that he would say a lover from Algeria with a visa problem was not his kind of issue, and promptly show me the door.

Thankfully, when I met Barry, he welcomed me warmly into his domain with a kind smile. I relaxed almost immediately. He laughed when I told him some of the answers on our failed visa that we had submitted. But he seemed interested – he wanted to know a lot more about how we met, and asked if I could show him any kind of verification of our communication. He was delighted when I told him I had saved every single landline and mobile telephone statement from the last seven months, as well as all the emails we had sent each other. I had them all hoarded on my computer.

"You've done the right thing by saving them," he said sincerely, "can you print everything out and bring the paperwork to me next time we meet?"

I tried to remain calm at his reference to a 'next time'. He was going to help our case. I was getting somewhere. *Finally.*

"Yes of course I can," I said in earnest.

"They'll be especially useful to show the Home Office as proof you two are in a relationship," he emphasised. "I would also need to read the full details of the entire failed visa."

My heart sank.

"But we don't have the original application form, and we didn't keep a copy," I said glumly.

"If I take on your case," he continued, "I can legally apply to the Home Office to retrieve the original application. That way I can fully understand your situation and see the mistakes you made."

I let out a sigh of relief. How could I have been so nervous on arrival? I now felt completely at ease with this charming man who clearly wanted to do all he could to help. I shook his hand, thanked him several times more than necessary, and left his office. I felt so much lighter as I walked back to the tube station, stepping over my own puke by the vegetable stall on the way.

On my second visit to his office a few days later, Barry stared in amazement at the two-inch-thick wad of paper I set down on the desk in front of him. I had printed out all the emails we had sent to each other, in chronological order. I also handed over several months of telephone and mobile phone statements, confirming we had been in touch regularly, as well as a few photographs of the two of us on holiday.

"Very well done," Barry said, chuckling, as he flipped through the stack of pages before him, "this is all extremely useful".

He recommended that the best way to secure a visa was to indicate Angelo was coming for an educational course in the UK.

"Well, I've already made an enquiry at a local language school," I explained. "I asked them if I could possibly enrol him in a course, providing he gets issued a visa."

Barry seemed impressed.

"That's really good news," he said, "plan ahead for next spring. I'll apply to the Home Office for the original application and go from there. If you have enrolled him already then we're ahead of the game."

A few days later, under Barry's guidance, after he received the original visa application from the British Consulate in Tunis, and telling the whole truth, Angelo and I began to fill in the new visa application form.

Once again, Angelo planned the long journey to the British Consulate in Tunis. This time he was clutching his second – final, we hoped – visa application. He was standing in the same place he'd visited just a few weeks earlier, but this time he was holding a more promising document in his hand.

After a terribly long wait, and another nerve-wracking interview, he was told he would have to come back the next day to find out the results. Meanwhile, back in Saltdean, I had practically chewed my fingers to the bone waiting for news this time. I couldn't shake the horrible, Groundhog Day feeling that we had been here before.

But then early the next morning – Algerian time – my ecstatic, exceedingly smiley man was screeching down the phone with such palpable excitement that I could barely make out any coherent speech.

We had done it. He finally had a visa.

The relief, the sheer joy in his voice was amazing. He was euphoric. The endless planning and sleepless nights to get him here had finally paid off. He was granted a nine-month student visa to come to England. Success at last.

A very happy Algerian left Tunis clutching his visa documents, then headed on the long journey home to tell his family and friends he would soon be leaving for England.

His family were shocked, yet delighted, that their son was starting a new chapter in his life. They could see he was happy. I know he explained to his parents where his new home in England was, and who he would be staying with, but I had no idea if they questioned him about my role in this exodus from Algeria. Surely, they must have wondered who I was.

**

Early on a January morning in 2006, I was pacing the arrivals hall at Heathrow Airport. I'm always early for meetings and appointments, and this was, of course, no exception – in my anxious anticipation I'd been awake since dawn.

My phone was in my hand ready to take the first picture of Angelo on UK soil. As I waited for a glimpse of him, I began to think of the events that had brought the two of us to this point. How we first met on a gay dating site, the problems entering Tunisia, the awful visa scenario we experienced with no resolution at hand, the endless journeys he took to obtain any kind of visa, and the sadness of being thousands of miles apart in the process.

There were sceptical people who couldn't understand our relationship and asked why I was inviting a young man from North Africa to live with me in England in the first place. They never thought for a moment that he was a true lover and life companion. I did hear a couple of negative jibes, meant as jokes, said to me over the previous weeks: "He's after your money mate"; "He wants a free ride here". (As I'm not a wealthy actor able to splash cash about that clearly was out of the question.)

Statistically, I am sure relationships that begin in this way on the internet often do not work. Perhaps the odds of our partnership working had been low, or non-existent. But here was proof to those sceptics who judged us or questioned our reasons for being together – we made it happen. He was on his way.

Besides, I knew everyone would love Angelo once they met him. I knew they would understand why I had jumped over several dozen hurdles to get him here. I could honestly say that it felt like the most natural thing for me to be doing, standing in the middle of the airport waiting for my lover of ten months from a faraway land to arrive to take him to my home by the seaside.

I waited with bated breath until I saw the unloading baggage sign light up. I continued pacing around, watching the first few visitors make their way out of the customs area. Then I spotted him, in a line of passengers, coming through the customs exit dragging a silly number of suitcases – a sight that would become a well-remembered image.

On my phone, I filmed the first couple of minutes of his arrival. I still have the clip. He walked towards me, laughing when he realised that I was filming him.
"Hello, you, and welcome to England!" I said with such joy in my voice.
We hugged in full view of anyone who wanted to watch. Finally, he was here with his big beaming smile and his arms around me in the middle of the arrivals hall.

We walked arm in arm, giggling and chatting, on the way back to the airport car park.
"I've not had a smoke since the Algiers airport," he said as he urgently pulled a cigarette from his jacket pocket and puffed away while we loaded his luggage into the car boot. He would have to get used to how antisocial smoking had become in the UK – there were no such things as 'no smoking' signs in Algiers.

Our maiden car journey down the motorways to East Sussex was an extraordinary feeling for us both. The M25 motorway is not usually the most romantic place, but that day, travelling along it together, touching hands and chatting away, it certainly was. After the turmoil and angst of the last couple of months, we were sitting side by side, in my old car, on our way to my house in Saltdean.

I felt my life was changing for the better as we entered Brighton.

"The sea, I can see the sea!" Angelo exclaimed excitedly as we headed straight down through the city. This section of the journey always thrills me, driving along the coast road, past the Brighton marina, towards home. I love coming back to Brighton at the best of times, but with Angelo beside me, it was even more magical. Living in the middle of Algeria – neighbouring the Sahara Desert – a view of the sea was not as common an occurrence for him as it was for me. Now he was seeing the English Channel for the first time.

As we pulled into my driveway, I worried about what he would think of my very British house. I knew that his parents' home was a vast apartment in an exclusive block of flats that his dad owned. My mid-century bungalow was nothing like the buildings he was used to seeing, so would he feel at home?

We unloaded his luggage and walked the pathway to my front door. Flossie was waiting to greet us inside the large central hallway.

"Hello pussy cat," he said happily, giving her a loving scratch behind her ear. He laughed as Dottie and George, my other two cats, trotted over to assess him. He was a cat person, thankfully.

"We have a lovely black cat at home that my mum and I love. We call her Minou," he said, while my cats circled his ankles.

I had never heard the name before, so I asked him what it meant. He said it was roughly translated into English as 'Minge'. He seemed puzzled at my stunned expression and the following fit of hysterics. I'm not sure his mum understood the English meaning.

When I showed him around the kitchen at the end of the hallway, I had another immediate worry: how could I expect him to like my British home cooking? It's not that I'm a bad cook at all – I love to cook for other people. But I was concerned his palate would test my cooking ability.

"Your mum is a particularly good home cook, you told me," I said as I watched him familiarise himself with the cupboards and cooking areas.

"Oh, yes. There were five of us at home and she cooked for us every day," he said proudly. I had a lot to live up to. Months later, once he was settled, he would phone his mum to ask for her recipes, continuing to chat with her as he cooked. Expensive long phone calls, but as a result, the dishes were delicious. He would cook a huge variety of Algerian dishes, much to the delight of our dinner guests who came to eat, followed by desserts he learned from his big brother, a trained French pâtissier.

I had a successful, happy life with my late partner Robert. This new chapter was going to be totally different from living with an English actor. There was no guarantee that this arrangement would work, but after the mammoth task to get him here, we were ready to give it our best shot.

CHAPTER SIXTEEN

"Can you take me to visit a gay bar one evening?" Angelo asked, soon after settling into my home. "I've never been inside one. I want to know for myself what it's like."
He knew there were piles of them in Brighton. In Algeria, there are no such gay venues. There are gay people living there, male and female, of course, but they cannot be open with their sexuality in their daily lives. They keep their true selves discreetly hidden from the public, for fear of persecution, or a prison sentence. So, of course, he was interested in at least sampling what was on offer in the gay capital of the UK.

I'd been to gay bars in London a few times in my younger years, mostly to dance with friends to extremely loud disco music. But as I got older and moved to the coast, the pull of the dancefloor had long since left me.

That night, I took him to visit a couple of places in town simply to show him what it was like inside. We ordered drinks in one of the bars and stood awkwardly in the gloom with music thumping in our ears. It wasn't a nightclub or anything extraordinary; it didn't exactly have the disco atmosphere I suspected he had hoped for. It was just a regular bar, a simple pub on a Tuesday with a mostly homosexual clientele. Perhaps I should have picked a better spot or waited for a busier day. But, as I said, my – short-lived –clubbing days were behind me, so I was rather out of the loop.

"This is so dreary to me," he said glumly, making no effort to conceal his disappointment. "Is this what people usually do in here? Stand or sit in this dark place and drink beer?"
I laughed at his ill-concealed disdain. He clearly couldn't understand the attraction – nor could I, truthfully. The drab ordinariness of the décor did not thrill him; I'm sure he must have imagined gay bars like those he saw in movies – trendy and chic,

illuminated by disco balls and strobe lights. There was no such glitz and glamour here.

We finished our drinks pretty sharpish and made a swift exit. Unsurprisingly, he never asked to go 'out' again.

**

After living together for a week, Angelo started his course at the St Giles language school. Although having an English Language degree already meant he was way ahead of the classes he attended, so he sometimes was rather bored.

"I feel like I am treading water or wasting my time there," he remarked one evening over dinner.

"You know the deal with the solicitor was to attend the college to secure the visa in the first place," I explained.

He grumbled a little, but he knew it was part of the deal.

Thankfully, the course was filled with many other international pupils who were starting at the same time, so he quickly began to make friends, which made him a lot happier. I was glad too – I knew it was important for him to meet new people that had nothing to do with me. The people he had met socially, so far, were my older British friends, although he fitted in very well with them. Every one of my friends I introduced him to welcomed him warmly into the fold. It was a thrill for me to watch their reactions as I first introduced such a handsome, charming new partner to them.

He had gladly adopted his new name of Angelo – he used it on all his official documents, even his payslips. It suited him perfectly, given that people had always assumed he was Italian.

"It's possible I was conceived in Italy anyway," he said one day.

"Why would you think that?" I asked.

"Well, my parents did go on holiday there many months before I was born, so it's very possible."

I chuckled. He certainly looked as though he had stepped off a runway in Milan – his stylish clothes were far trendier than the local English men his age where we lived. His style was different, and he was proud of it. It was a joy showing my partner around the town and watching passers-by react to his eye-catching, very un-English dress sense.

"How I would have loved to have attended university here," Angelo said wistfully, on several occasions, as I showed him the sights of his new city. He saw the freedom students experienced in Brighton, and a more international, mixed group of young people in the city than he had in Oran. And his taste-buds were tantalised by the fashion consciousness of the young people and their dress sense and style from all over the world.

He was fascinated by the stylish boutiques in Brighton, but he practically went berserk when we visited places like Liberty, Selfridges, and even John Lewis in London. The whole of Oxford Street was like a kind of paradise to him.

On our shopping trips to London and days out perusing The Lanes in Brighton, we would talk endlessly about Angelo's immediate future after his language course finished. We both knew his talent and interests lay in fashion design. He learned that well-established fashion designers – such as Denise Ho, Julien Macdonald, and BIBA founder Barbara Hulanicki – had first trained in Brighton, and this really encouraged him to follow in their footsteps. So, we started to discuss the possibility of him applying to university here in the autumn.

In the meantime, he needed to work and earn some money and was reminded of the time he was on a plane journey from Algiers airport to the British Consulate in Tunis, Algeria, holding his second visa application form, he met on board a couple of girls whom he befriended. They were both Air Algérie cabin crew, and like him, they were en route to the British Consulate to obtain their UK visas.

The three had a lot in common obviously and decided to stay in the same cheap hotel in Tunis on that first evening before visiting the Consulate early the next morning. During dinner together, the girls talked of boyfriends they were dating, and one said: "I have a boyfriend who lives in England, he owns a restaurant in a seaside town called Brighton". Angelo couldn't believe his ears: "That's the city where I will live and go to college, if I get this visa". The girl immediately encouraged Angelo to contact her boyfriend after he arrived: "He may be able to give you a job", she said excitedly.

The details and phone number of the man were written down and it was up to him to find the restaurant owner when he successfully arrived in England. What a stroke of luck he thought, meeting these girls on the same plane. Once he obtained his student visa and was established in Brighton, he made it his mission to find this man.

Arriving in Brighton he sought out the restaurant owner and was indeed given a job working as a waiter in what he thought would be a perfect one with an Algerian restaurant owner. But the place was a shambles, there was no training for the mostly foreign students, and the regular staff helped themselves to his wages when he wasn't looking. So, naturally, he made a quick getaway, but not before he accidentally dropped a tray of champagne cocktails over the surprised customers.

After that, he was able to pick up a few weekend shifts working for a catering company that serviced racecourses around Brighton and wider Sussex. He enjoyed the work, and he quickly made friends. He also learned silver service waitering, something he had never tried his hand at before, but was rather good at.

He was a busy boy during his first months in Brighton, studying at the language school during the week, and working shifts at the racecourse on the weekends. On top of that, in his free time from college, he planned his application for university, which called for a design portfolio complete with fabric samples to showcase his talent. He worked on his designs in the evenings after college or when he was not working at the racecourse. Any sceptics who thought he came to England for an easy life were clearly wrong. He worked his bum off.

Luckily, he had brought a rather large portfolio of his designs and drawings with him from Algeria, some he had created during his time studying fashion in Lyon some years before. Looking through his past work of intricately detailed designs of gowns, I realised that he truly had an outstanding talent. But he was determined to update this portfolio to be more current.

We travelled to London to visit a collection of fabric shops which were conveniently squeezed into one small area of the city, on Brewer Street in Soho. We probably visited every shop in the street searching for bits of material he thought appropriate to accompany each of his designs. Unsurprisingly, the shop owners were charmed by him almost instantly, so they happily gave him cut-offs of whatever fabric he asked for to enhance the creations in his portfolio.

His completed presentation for his university application was inspired. Scraps of materials from Brewer Street were pinned to each design, so his portfolio was bulging. I was enormously proud and full of admiration for the work involved. Beaming with joy, he proudly handed over his high-class designs, desperately hoping his dreams would soon become a reality.

But there was another hurdle to jump before that dream could be realised: his present student visa would run out in October, which meant applying once again to the British Consulate in Tunis for the next one. Yes, this was months away, but his visa situation was always at the back of our minds. It was a nightmare of a journey for him to look forward to, from Brighton to Tunis, and back again.

The 'indefinite leave to remain' visa status was the ultimate one to obtain, which would keep him in the country permanently. We began to query if there was a way to get the ultimate status more quickly. One solution to establish a more secure base together in this country was unconventional, and, at the time, still rather unheard of.

A civil partnership.

We had never thought of such a thing before, especially as same-sex ceremonies were very new, having only come into existence in the UK less than six months before. But with our lives flourishing well together as a couple, it seemed to make perfect sense for us to make the relationship permanent on paper. And if doing so it made a difference in securing his status in this country, then we were damn well going to try it.

So, we made an appointment with the local registrar. I remember that day at the town hall so clearly, grinning like Cheshire cats as we filled in the paperwork and handed it over. We were both so thrilled at the prospect of doing such a grown-up thing together. What a year it had been.

Our future together looked promising.

CHAPTER SEVENTEEN

The earliest couples in England and Wales (same-sex or otherwise) could proceed with a civil partnership ceremony was late in December 2005. Our ceremony was planned to take place in May 2006, so we must have been in the first batch of ceremonies in the East Sussex area. We would have loved to have had a summer ceremony, but those dates had been booked up by eager couples who got there first. So, we were set to be legally recognised life partners only a few months after Angelo touched down on English soil.

The hunt then was on around all the jewellery shops in Brighton for a set of rings for the big day.

"I know we both want simple rings, but can we have some sort of diamond in the ring?" Angelo pleaded.

"You mean a diamond like Elizabeth Taylor would wear?" I said jokingly. "I don't think so." Unfortunately for my soon-to-be partner, I wasn't on that sort of actor's salary.

Still, we wandered The Lanes to find something cheap and simple with the smallest diamond in the centre.

We only asked two close friends to be our witnesses during the ceremony. There were no other guests invited to the town hall. We had little or no money available to have a decent celebration with our friends – we had only enough to buy the rings and, of course, decent outfits for us to wear on the day. A reception afterwards was out of the question.

We explained to our dear friends, Tony and Christine Adams, who lived in the next street, that we couldn't afford a big get-together, so our ceremony would be a low-key affair, followed by a quiet drink in a pub near the town hall afterwards. Tony Adams was a good friend I had known for years, having understudied him in my first West End show, *The Boyfriend*. They had met Angelo many times for dinners, at theirs or my place, and they both adored him.

"Under *no* circumstances will that happen," Christine said firmly, without missing a beat. "Tony and I will give you both a party and a reception here in our home to celebrate. Ask a few friends."

I pulled Christine into a big hug as I felt my stiff upper lip begin to quiver. I couldn't quite believe my ears. It was such a generous gift. Their announcement meant we could invite a few people to attend the town hall ceremony and the reception in their home afterwards. At such short notice, there was a chance only a handful of people would be free to come at all, but I managed to round up a small group at the last minute.

My agent, Lesley, came down from London, appearing at our house incredibly early in the morning, looking gorgeous. We were already suited and booted for the occasion when she arrived, so the three of us sat around drinking coffee, chatting, and smoking. But our nattering was interrupted by the post landing with a thud on the hall floor.

I picked it up and rifled through the letters as I walked back to the living room, pausing when I spotted an official-looking, weighty envelope addressed to Angelo, with UCAS printed on the front. We all knew it was the result of the application from Brighton University. No one wanted to open it, least of all Angelo, so the letter got handed around between us until Lesley took charge, opened it, and read the opening lines out loud: "You've been accepted to start the design course at Brighton University this coming September!" she said with a squeal. "Well done my dear."

Angelo leapt up from the sofa with a wonderfully theatrical gasp, almost dousing our wedding outfits in hot coffee. He was thrilled – we all were. What joy, what a time to receive this letter on the day we were having our civil partnership. I cannot quite articulate the euphoria we felt.

That morning, before we left for the registry office, I contacted my solicitor who helped secure the visa. I wanted to tell him the news of our ceremony, and of Angelo's acceptance letter from university arriving on the same day.

"Many congratulations to both of you!" he said, sounding incredibly pleased. "Especially to Angelo for the place at university."

He seemed truly happy for us. I asked if having a civil partner would help with the next visa. He said it probably would. Then I told him we were having our honeymoon in two days' time, back to Tunisia where we first met the year before.

"In that case," he said, "as you're both in the vicinity, it might be a good opportunity to go to the capital, he might be eligible for the indefinite leave to remain status. Why not try for the next one?"

So, nervous but elated, Angelo and I were standing in my hallway, smartly dressed, waiting for the taxi to take us to the town hall when the phone rang. It was my big brother John. I was puzzled as our chats together were usually at the weekend, so a mid-week call was unusual. The timing was extraordinary, particularly as he knew nothing of our intentions that morning.

Sadly, I never asked my family to come to the ceremony. Aside from the fact that getting them down to Brighton at short notice was prohibitive, I had not yet told them about this man in my life. When Robert and I became a serious item and moved in together, the situation with our family was so easy. They accepted that he was a part of my life without me ever having to come out or define what our relationship was. Of course, Robert died over a decade before I met Angelo, but my family all adored him. I had no idea what they would think about a new person entering my life, so I decided not to say anything. But the universe, it seemed, had other plans.

"Hello, how are you?" John asked pleasantly.

I paused to reply.

"I'm fine... is there anything wrong?" I was expecting him to tell me of a family disaster at home.

"No, I'm just asking if anything's happening down there."

What a bizarre thing to say, today of all days. I was so taken by surprise and rather dumbstruck. Then I suddenly felt I must explain to him exactly what was happening, and blurted out the whole scenario of meeting Angelo some months before, and that he had come to live with me in England. I gave him a potted version of the events of course, but he got the gist. The relief of explaining my present circumstances to John was uplifting. A huge weight fell off my shoulders.

"Congratulations!" he yelled, "I can't wait to ring Jackie and tell her."

What a revelation it was hearing my big brother happy and joyful for us both. Jackie, my lovely niece, rang almost immediately and gave us her congratulations as well. How unexpected all this was, and it happened moments before the taxi arrived to take us to the town hall. This was already such a joyful time for me, made even more glorious by my immediate family's blessing.

Was it fate that my brother should call that very morning? Yes, of course it was, it was meant to happen. It was no coincidence. I do not believe in them.

I asked Angelo, days before, if he would say anything to his parents about the town hall visit. This was not a good idea, he said. It was best for him to say nothing at all to his family, especially as they were only just getting used to the fact that he'd left the family nest to live in a new country many miles away. So, he never did mention this special day we'd planned for a civil partnership. I wondered if they would even know such a ceremony between a same-sex couple was possible in this country, let alone approve of such a thing. Probably not.

His family knew about me, my name, and that Angelo was living in my house. But did they fully understand our relationship? I doubted it. They never questioned him about it. I suppose to them I was his friend and landlord. They were happy, I believed, that he had a comfortable house to live in, pleased he attended the language course, and had a part-time job. So, I'm sure they had no real problem with his living arrangements. Realistically, they would hardly assume the truth of the situation.

Angelo phoned home all the time, particularly to speak with his mum. It was clear he had a good relationship with his parents – he always sounded happy when he talked to them. Occasionally, I heard my name mentioned in the conversation, but in what context, I never knew. I spoke to his mum a couple of times on the landline when she rang. My French was stilted but I managed a brief, pleasant chat with her. So at least I was not an alien. At the start of our relationship, she mildly questioned him about me and even as the months went by, she didn't pry.

Most of the guests coming to our civil ceremony were old friends of mine, but they had only met Angelo a handful of times by then. Thankfully, he had invited a few friends from college which meant the event was not going to be completely overrun with my vocal theatrical pals.

One of those attending was my dear, fabulous friend Elizabeth Edmiston, who had introduced me to my fairy godmother, Michael Cashman, months ago. How mad it was to think that this day was a direct knock-on effect of my conversation with dear Lizzie. It was entirely through her help that we were standing in that town hall at all, professing our true love for each other in front of our friends. I was more than delighted that she and Erica were with us to celebrate – they were a joyful addition to our special day.

Lizzie had been rather ill at the time, but she was no less determined to make the journey to Brighton. She arrived wearing a rather wild hat covered with a meadow's worth of flowers that she had bought in La Rue des Juifs in Paris. Classy Lizzie was enormously proud to wear it on this occasion.

Our original group were two singers, my friends Paul and Paula (not a double act), plus the two of us, making four. Thanks to Christine and Tony, we were joined by 12 other loving friends to help us celebrate.

The celebrant was a beautifully spoken lady, a wonderful orator. Every loving word she delivered to us was heartfelt. Angelo and I beamed with joy as we exchanged our cheap, but lovingly selected, rings, signing the register while our favourite jazz singer, Stacey Kent's voice sang *I'm Putting All My Eggs In One Basket* through the sound system. Then, in a picture-perfect moment, the two of us emerged from the grand front doors of the town hall, dwarfed by the magnificent, fluted columns on either side of us. We laughed in delight as we were met with cheers and a flurry of biodegradable confetti before we all made our way to Chez Adams in Saltdean.

The spread that Christine and Tony put on put every single one of my dinner parties to shame. Christine, an amazing cook, had gone to town with a sumptuous table of goodies, and she made sure the champagne was flowing – there wasn't an empty glass in the house. Tony was a magnificent host and delivered some exceedingly kind words about me being his oldest male friend (I hoped he was referring to our relationship and not my age). After everyone had eaten, and with their glasses full, I said a few nervous words of thank you to our guests. It's funny that, as an actor, I have no trouble delivering lines onstage to hundreds of strangers, yet, in such an intimate setting, I found it difficult to express just how overjoyed and filled with gratitude I was to have such generous friends, and such a wonderful partner by my side.

More old pals were meeting Angelo for the first time, each of them marvelling over what a charming, handsome, young man he was. Dear friends congratulated us for the entirety of the afternoon (the free-flowing champagne meant that some repeated the same congratulations several times over the course of the night). One of my mates had brought his video camera and was asking our guests to say a few words for Angelo and me to watch back later. When it was the turn of my dear friend Helen and her fella, Helen – who was pissed by this point – spoke sincerely to the camera about how delighted she was for the happy couple, wishing Andrew and me a wonderful life together.

"Who the bloody hell is Andrew?!" someone squealed. Of course, screams of laughter ensued, and poor Helen was mortified.

There was such a great feeling of love surrounding us both, and I knew everyone who was with us that day knew this was a genuine love affair, not just some sort of marriage of convenience.

The rest of the day passed in a blissful haze. Although at one point I was sitting in the garden – it was a pleasantly balmy May evening – chatting with an old friend, Maps Woolcott, when I caught sight of my ring finger.

"Oh my God!" I gasped, "the diamond in my ring has fallen out – I've only been wearing it for the last three hours!" I was horrified. This ring, the symbol of our partnership, hung on my finger, naked. I hoped to God that this wasn't some sort of horrible omen for our future.

"This relationship is doomed already, dear!" Maps remarked, as though he had read my mind. He was laughing his head off. "You can't go on a 'homo-moon' with no diamond on your finger!"

Thankfully, his cackling was infectious, and peals of laughter burst from both of us. I guess 'you get what you pay for' applies to cheap rings, too.

When the group started to disperse in the evening, we slowly meandered home down the hill to our house on the next street, overwhelmed but elated by the day's events, and the knowledge that we had our names in print, side by side, announcing that we were an official couple.

CHAPTER EIGHTEEN

Our second visit to Tunisia was off to a much more relaxing start than our first, although the impending visit to the British Consulate clouded what otherwise should have been a sensational honeymoon, and added a level of anxiety surely not felt by most newlyweds. But, we were intent on enjoying some well-needed rest after the excitement of our civil partnership and the chaos of getting everything ready for our trip two days later.

The hotel, in Hammamet, not far from The Sinbad where we had visited my dear friend Paul almost a year before, was a quiet one in a great location. We had a large suite and balcony overlooking more perfumed gardens, right by the sea and a walkable distance to another large souk, which allowed for endless shopping trips to find unusual gifts to take home to our friends. What an extraordinary circle of events this was, returning to such a fabulous place as a couple – it was a perfect spot for our first holiday as legally recognised partners.

Two days after we arrived, as we were getting ready to head to the Consulate, I was in a state of utter panic.
"Have you got all the documents? Nothing's missing?" I asked cautiously.
Angelo quashed my nerves by producing a mass of paperwork from his day bag. "Look, here's the passport, the application form, our bank statements, and of course the letter from the university," he said calmly.
I imagined the letter declaring he had a place waiting for him at university in September would make all the difference for him qualifying for permanent status in the UK.

The queue at the Consulate was enormous when we arrived. People from thousands of miles away were there with hopes of obtaining a visa to enter the UK, so the waiting room was crowded with rows upon rows of occupied chairs. We filed in together, took our numbered tickets, and begrudgingly waited our turn.

After an age, Angelo was called over by a stern-looking official and ushered into a glass-panelled booth. I nervously watched as he faced another stone-faced member of the Consulate staff. From where I was sitting, I couldn't hear their voices clear enough to know exactly what they were saying, but I could make out a lot of mumbling and head nodding. I took this as a good sign. Angelo handed over the papers and then they asked him to return to me in the waiting area while the officer scrutinised the documents for a while.

"I think that went well..." he started to say, but before he could finish his sentence I was beckoned over by the same man.

"What does he want to see me for?" I asked, puzzled, as I made my way to the booth.

This we were not expecting – it wasn't me who was applying for a visa, after all – so I was decidedly nervous.

The interviewer held our civil partnership document in his hands. He asked endless questions about our relationship, examined the visa application line by line, then went back to asking me more – rather invasive, I thought – questions about our relationship. The whole process was anxiety-inducing, having a complete stranger interrogate you about some of the most intimate details of your love life.

The questions were to trip me up, I guessed, in case either of us was lying about our relationship. I was terrified. I felt like a criminal, as though I had committed some terrible deed. Was I on trial here? Usually, I am at ease and upfront about talking about myself. I never hide anything of my persona, I'm too much of an open book for that. But now I felt I was hiding something I ought to have been ashamed of. It was a weird feeling, certainly not one I wanted to experience again.

A short while later, I was dismissed by the officer and asked to sit back with Angelo in the waiting area. The interviewer disappeared for quite some time, taking the documents away to be scrutinised further, I assumed, somewhere way out of our sight.

We waited for what felt like hours, oblivious as to why there was such a delay, or whether the visit was going well, or not. We sat in silence for most of the time, not quite sure what to say to each other.

Our interviewer eventually returned with the wad of paperwork we had given to him, and Angelo was called back into the booth again for a second, longer interview. I waited and watched, nauseous, with the same feeling of guilt sweeping over me again. The palms of my hands were drenched with sweat. It may have been Angelo's third visit to the same Consulate, but I could tell it wasn't any easier for him this time around, even with me there. It's not something you get used to.

The result of our interrogation was not a positive one.
"We have been refused on two grounds," Angelo said flatly when he returned to me with an ashen face. "First, my present visa has not yet expired. This means I'm okay to return at the end of our week and remain in the UK for a few more months."
This we both knew anyway.
"Secondly, they can see from our bank statements that we don't jointly have the £9,000 a foreign student needs for the first year's fee at university."
We both fully understood the university fee was to be paid well before September, and to honour this, if we couldn't scrape that amount together beforehand, my plan was to get a loan against my house, well before the payment was needed.

Each with a face like a slapped arse, we left the Consulate and stood in the sunny street, on the same spot Angelo had stood twice before, facing a similar outcome.
"I'm devastated," he said glumly. "I thought we had covered all areas to make it foolproof." I could tell he was close to tears. As was I, truth be told.
"I know," I said. "It's my fault we included that letter from the university." I thought it would help our case, not hinder it.

It seemed we had blown it. And the big drag at the back of both of our minds was the fact that, when he inevitably applied for a new visa, he would have to make the arduous journey back to this same Consulate, yet again. But I knew our disappointment had to be short-lived; our melancholic mood had to lift, there and then.

"Look, Angelo, we are in Tunisia on our honeymoon," I said, "you still have a few months left on the visa in your pocket, so all is not doom and gloom. We can fly home safely, together, after the holiday."

"Yes, I know, you're right," Angelo admitted with a sigh. "Let's go back to our hotel, have a drink, and try and relax. I'm totally shattered."

So, once we shook off the foul form that threatened to ruin our romantic getaway, we got straight to enjoying more fragrant, temperate Tunisian evenings together, albeit amidst a much friendlier crowd of mixed nationalities this time around. Thankfully, it turned out to be a terrific week, all things considered, with lots of time to swim, sun ourselves, and smoke local cigarettes on the beach under our hotel's gaudy umbrellas.

We loved it there. *Vive le Tunisie*.

We left Africa feeling refreshed, but back in Brighton, we faced more disappointing news. Angelo's present visa wouldn't cover the starting dates of the university course, and he couldn't begin the term without a new visa in place. There was no option other than for him to write to the university and withdraw from the place he so desperately wanted to take. It was a devastating decision. The design course, after all, could have changed his life. His painstakingly crafted portfolio, which was bursting at the seams with intricate designs, was now of no use. I was desperately upset watching his dreams evaporate in the letter he wrote.

In the autumn, as his language course at college was behind him, and his latest visa was expiring, again, he made the trek back to Tunis. Ahead of him were the joys of collecting that numbered ticket in the long queue at the British Consulate, with yet another application in hand.

This would be his fourth visit in two years. I tried not to dwell on the irony that the amount of money we spent on all his trips back and forth to Tunis would have covered a whole year's university fees.

Luckily, it was his last one.

I answered the phone to a breathless Angelo, who was barely able to contain his excitement: "I've got the big one, indefinite leave to remain!"

He returned to England elated, triumphant, and for good. At long last.

CHAPTER NINETEEN

After three years together, our relationship had grown solid – how quickly and blissfully the time had passed. We were both earning money: Angelo was now working regularly in a Brighton boutique, and I had the odd acting job. In those days, I also had my own website where I sold collectable vinyl records. I collected these, bit by bit, over decades, from junk shops, and car boot sales. Providing they were of good quality and desirable to collectors, I bought them and sold them on. It was a way to earn cash on the side that I was rather good at; I had sold and exported my records to all parts of the world.

We were living together happily. I adored the home we had created together, as did all of our friends, whom we often entertained for dinner. But despite how secure and content we were together, I could tell that Angelo wanted more from his life in the UK.

"I've been thinking," he said one day over breakfast, "even though I can't be kicked out of the country, I'd like to have an even more permanent status here. I'd like to become a British citizen."

"Really? That's wonderful!" I said, delighted. "Why not do it, it should make life easier at the airports when we go on holiday."

Over the last few years, poor Angelo's life seemed to have been consumed by application forms and interviews. Although this time, things went a lot more quickly.

The ceremony was to take place in a large, grand room at Hove Town Hall in 2009. It's a rather imposing, brutalist, glass-fronted building, definitely not as pretty as Brighton Town Hall, where we had our civil partnership ceremony three years before. But still, it was a lovely day – the sun was splitting the sky when we arrived, which we hoped was a good omen. We were accompanied by one of Angelo's girlfriends, who came to witness the ceremony. She was Swedish and was fascinated to see what happened at an event of this sort.

Under the watchful eye of an enormous and imposing portrait of Queen Elizabeth II, leaning on a huge easel, several rows of seats were set up for the vast number of applicants applying for citizenship, who were accompanied by their families and friends. People of all ages, creeds, and religions from all corners of the world filled the room; applicants from Uzbekistan to Australia and most countries in between were there applying for British citizenship. It was a marvellously exciting thing to witness and be part of, perhaps the most special ceremony that I have attended in all my life.

There was a welcome speech from the council dignitary officiating, and then each recipient was asked to recite collectively their allegiance to the Crown and the Queen. As the Queen was also the head of the Church of England, recipients who were Christians recited a few religious lines. Those of a different religion had slightly different wording for their allegiance. This applied to Angelo of course.

It was then the officiant's duty to call out every single person's name and the country they originated from to come forward to receive, from him, their document of British citizenship. There was much applause and cheering from every quarter of the room as each person came forward to the podium. The officiant shook each person by the hand and then posed for official photographs to be taken with each recipient. Naturally, I rushed to the presentation area to be in the picture when Angelo's name was called. There I stood, immensely proud, with my grinning civil partner, who was now an official Brit.

Soon after the ceremony, Angelo and I began to talk about what our future would look like together. After being forced to give up on his university dream some years before, Angelo had started sketching again. Only now his drawings changed from couture gowns to intricate sketches of leather handbags of all descriptions.

I watched him drawing, sometimes for hours, as I was so intrigued by the work he could produce. I was delighted – relieved, honestly – that he had, at last, rediscovered his passion. In fact, it seemed he was now more determined than ever to break into the industry. He constantly scoured the internet for the latest trends, and I would accompany him to research the new season leather goods in the big stores in London. The price ladies pay for a named designer bag, to me, was ludicrous, although I understood why Angelo wanted a slice of the designer handbag pie. It was an immense, but potentially lucrative, industry that he wanted to enter, and I wanted to encourage him in any way I could.

His basic idea was that we could use his talent to draw high-end designs, then search for a way to have prototypes made and find a market for them. It was a fantasy at this moment, but we knew there was a possibility that we could turn it into our reality.

My acting career had been successful and fulfilling, but for a long time, I had felt the need to do something different with my life apart from theatre and television shows. For a little while, at least. Besides, I knew I could always go back to the theatre world if I wanted to – the performer's passion still ran through my veins.

I liked the idea of being involved with my partner in a business venture. The two of us working in tandem seemed to fit. I knew I had a flair for business, something I was good at apart from my professional theatre work. So, this venture we had in mind, using my partner's designs and my business knowledge, seemed ideal.

"Would you come with me, if I wanted to visit a leather trade show I've seen advertised?" Angelo asked me one day when trawling through the internet. The trade show was to be held in Istanbul, Turkey; the arena was in a vast building on the outskirts of the city, specially designed for business enterprises. He really believed it would be a great event to attend, and I totally agreed.

Nothing ventured, nothing gained. Plus, I would never say no to a chance of winter sun.

We flew to Istanbul in November 2009. It was also the first time Angelo could use his new maroon British passport which, for him, was a huge excitement. Zooming past the bustling streets in a taxi, we caught a glimpse of the infamous Blue Mosque rising between the buildings of this amazing, sprawling city that straddled the Bosporus. I knew Angelo wanted to visit the mosque – although he never visited the ones back home in England – as did I. But, sadly, as our time in Istanbul was so limited, all we got to see was its beautiful exterior.

The trade fair was huge, much bigger than Angelo or I had imagined. We stood in an enormous, modern foyer with staircases that led to different levels above us. Signs were everywhere to indicate the various areas of interest, but still, we had no clue where to begin.

Angelo tentatively explained the reason for our visit to a few different stallholders, but there was only a smattering of English speakers here and there, so talking to everyone we met was not easy. Although he was able to pick up most Arabic dialects, Turkish was not easy for Angelo to grasp. He tried to ask questions of anyone who might look like they were interested in why we were there, but it didn't take long for us to realise we were completely out of our depth, and out of place. We had no idea what to do. We had travelled all this way for nothing, it seemed.

Luckily, we stumbled upon a man with a small display of leather goods who spoke a little English. He seemed interested in why on earth we were there at all (I'll admit, I had begun to wonder the same). He took time to listen to Angelo, before taking a grubby scrap of paper from his pocket and drawing a little, rather vague, map of what seemed to be a market area. He assured us that there we should find people who would help us with our quest. We were intrigued.

We took a taxi from the trade show arena right into the centre of Istanbul. How touching to be given directions by such a helpful old guy who didn't know us from Adam. We showed the taxi man the scrappy, hand-drawn map, and, miraculously, he knew exactly where to take us.

We were driven right into the middle of a labyrinth of tiny criss-crossing streets that housed hundreds of small, but clearly flourishing, businesses. They were dotted all over the place: shops huddled close together selling all kinds of fabrics and goods made of leather. There were craftsmen and women creating products in their shop fronts, their workplaces in clear view; materials of all colours and designs were hung in the tiny streets to entice customers inside.

"Oh boy! Where have we come to?" Angelo said excitedly.

It seemed we had landed slap-bang in the middle of Aladdin's cave. This was exactly what we were looking for.

Within minutes, Angelo spotted a display of beautiful designer handbags in one of the shop windows.

"They must be real, they can't be fakes," he said incredulously as he scrutinised the bags. I had no idea if they were real or not, but the shop was chic, glass-fronted, and immaculately clean, so it certainly didn't seem like a back street rip-off establishment.

Angelo's wonderment had caught the attention of the shop owner, who must have been curious as to why two strange men were examining her stock so intensely. Angelo explained, as best he could, in a couple of languages, why we were there. She seemed to understand, but then she indicated for us to stay in the shop as she reached for the telephone – maybe she was asking for security help to chuck us out.

Instead, moments later, we were greeted by a very friendly, very young, Congolese man, wearing old jeans, a scruffy T-shirt, and a dog collar. He was a Christian vicar.

"Hello," he said with a warm smile. "You're English?"

We nodded, rather perplexed.

"I've been asked to come and help the owner understand what you are looking for," he explained. "I'm an Anglican pastor, and I'm responsible for a large Anglican parish in the middle of Istanbul."

He told us he could speak fluent French and English. For Angelo, this man was a godsend, in all senses of the word. Now that the language problem wasn't a barrier, he was able to explain our business idea, why we were in this country, and what we were looking for.

We were chatting away with our new Anglican acquaintance when a larger, heavy-set, older-looking gentleman strode through the open door. The pastor greeted him warmly. To me, he was what I imagined a mafia boss would look like. It turned out he was, in fact, the father of the shop owner lady, and the daddy of this business we had stumbled on. The pastor explained to Daddy why we were there. Daddy looked extremely interested and told the pastor to invite us to join them all for lunch upstairs. This surprised and delighted us, not just because he looked like he might throw us out of the shop when he first arrived.

We climbed the stairs to the floor above the shop, to a space that seemingly doubled as the executive meeting room and the dining area. The five of us sat around a large boardroom table in the middle of this huge room, and suddenly five complete salad lunches and soft drinks appeared, as if from nowhere. The family and their pastor friend chatted between themselves as we ate; Angelo and I said very little to each other – our first day in Istanbul had us at a bit of a loss for words.

The pastor-slash-interpreter explained to the family the reasons we had visited Istanbul in the first place, and then he fired questions at Angelo and relayed the answers back to Daddy. It was established by then that Daddy was in charge of their leather business, and he owned his factory. He controlled all the products they made for the international market. He was rarely seen in the shop – that was his daughter's territory. He had arrived simply to see what was going on with the two off-season tourists. Clearly, Daddy was intrigued by our visit.

During all this time I hardly said a word, but sat by Angelo's side, trying to play my new role as 'Confident Businessman Number One'. If I was ever out of my depth appearing in a stage production, I could always fall back on my theatre experience and wing it. I hoped this skill in blagging would see me right.

It was clear that the pastor was the best possible link between us and any help, or perhaps even potential business, we could secure from the family. Finally, it looked like we were getting somewhere with our quest.

Lunch over and cleared away, Daddy, via the pastor, asked us if we would like to see his factory, on the outskirts of Istanbul, to which we responded with an eager, "Yes please!" Daddy drove a large, black car (again, very mafioso-like), and the pastor sat chatting in the front with him. Angelo and I sat in the back, bewildered by what we were experiencing, still saying very little to each other, apart from Angelo's repetition of, "This is amazing", under his breath.

We were ushered into the factory and on to the production floor where there was a double line of machinists working on various projects.
"Look at these guys working," Angelo said, in awe, as we were led down the line of machinists.
"This man is developing Prada design," the factory manager said in broken English, "the next one working on Gucci".
Neither Angelo nor I could believe it. Having examined their lookalikes in Selfridges, he had been so sure these bags were the real deal – they certainly were indistinguishable from replicas to my eyes.

Each worker had a design and clear measurements to follow for each section of the bag by their side. He showed us down both the lines of machinists, who were all men, explaining what designer they were copying. Angelo was wide-eyed throughout our tour. It was fascinating, for me too, to witness the skilled factory machinists at work.

"They sell their products only to the Far East, never to the western countries in Europe," the pastor told us as we left the factory to go back to their offices. He lowered his voice to continue: "The market they favoured was for the East because there are fewer restrictions on how genuine the named designer brands are there."

With the factory tour over, we exchanged various contact details so we could keep in touch. They talked again about Angelo returning later in the year to show them his designs in detail. From what we gathered that afternoon, there seemed to be a strong possibility they would produce his prototypes. We couldn't believe our luck. Then Daddy indicated to the pastor that he wanted to drive us back to our hotel. This was of course nowhere near their factory, but as we had no idea how to get back ourselves, we accepted gratefully. As they dropped us off in the hotel drive, we shook hands, hugged the pastor, and each of us said a very warm goodbye to each other.

Upon arriving back in our hotel room, we collapsed on to the freshly turned down bed, shattered, but jubilant.
"We never thought we would find such a family here, did we?" Angelo said with infectious delight. We thought we'd hit the jackpot.

Was meeting with this family a coincidence? No, it wasn't. I don't believe in them.

CHAPTER TWENTY

When we returned to Brighton, energy renewed, Angelo began to churn out design after design, spending most, if not all, of his free time sketching prototypes to take back to Istanbul. His plan was to return in a few weeks, this time alone. His solo visit made me slightly nervous, but this entire idea was his creation in the first place, and he had to make it work for himself. If the family could make these samples from his sketches, which we had some funds for, then we could be in business sometime soon.

The second meeting with the leather family was remarkably successful. Once again, the pastor was in attendance to help translate. They seemed to be keen to try and work something out with him after their machinists had thoroughly looked over his drawings. Then we would know if they could make samples quickly for us to really kick-start our business.

Upon returning to Brighton, both of us waited for a response with bated breath, but maintaining communication between the UK and Istanbul was not easy. The family only understood English if the interpreter was around, and he had his Anglican flock to look after in the city. Although he spent time helping the family with translations, he was not always on hand for a general chat whenever a phone call came from Brighton, so things there were moving at a slower pace than we imagined.

To help speed things along, Angelo recruited a Turkish girl who worked in a nearby sandwich bar who was able to phone for updates from time to time. But even still, we had to factor in the time difference, and the Islamic prayer times in the factory, which didn't exactly correspond with any regular working hours here. Angelo tried desperately to keep communication active but found it frustrating with no direct contact.

Just a glimpse of positive news was all he needed to encourage him to continue, but progress seemed to be at a standstill. The entire project started to slide away from us. News had filtered through that the shop in Istanbul was doing remarkably well, so the family had decided to open another shop in Ankara, the capital. With all their time and energy being used on their own new business venture, there was no time to help a young, unknown designer from Brighton.

This whole process had taken over months of Angelo's time. I knew how utterly frustrated and disappointed he was because I felt the same. Yet, I knew he would not give up easily. We both knew we could develop a thriving design business somehow; we just needed some help. So, we set about researching various government workshops where advice seminars were given for people, like us, intending to start a business. Luckily, there were several meetings held locally to help complete beginners when planning such a venture.

We were certainly beginners, and we were told regularly that plans like ours often failed before they could get off the ground. Many people started up a business with not enough background knowledge of what was ahead and failed in the first year. Brighton was (and still is) littered with such closures of small businesses, particularly coffee shops in The Lanes. We knew we were completely out of our depth, but we were determined to succeed.

Angelo started to search for other leather traders elsewhere. By now, he was working full-time in a trendy fashion boutique owned and run by two Jewish brothers who welcomed him with open arms. I held back theatre work as it would mean being away from home for weeks at a time, and I could make a reasonable amount of money selling my vinyl.

During our annual anniversary trip to Menorca in May of that year, I decided to sell my house in Saltdean. It felt like the natural next step for us as a couple, and it would help us kick-start our business – I could repay the small outstanding debt and buy another property mortgage-free. Then, when we needed it, I could raise a few grand on the new property.

Having established myself successfully in Saltdean, alone, I didn't think I would ever move from there. It held such a special place in my heart. So, selling up was a big decision, yes, but I was serious about my future with Angelo, and committed to supporting him in whatever way I could. A totally clean slate was needed to start any kind of business together. The excitement of planning this new venture overrode any sense of nostalgia that tied me to the house. Plus, choosing a home together was going to be a huge adventure for the both of us.

By the time we were back from Menorca, I placed the house on the market with a local estate agent in Rottingdean. Viewings for potential buyers began in earnest, which in turn meant we had to search quickly for a place to move to. I wasn't sure where to begin – I needed to make a profit selling up so I could buy the new home outright in order to give us the financial freedom to start our plans.

Selling houses, as anyone can tell you, is a tedious, boring, long-winded process. We had little time to focus on furthering our business, so our dream was presently on hold. To be honest, it was at a standstill.

For months on end, the house was kept immaculately tidy just in case anyone came around to look – this extended to the ginormous garden which, although quite spectacular and a definite selling point, was a pain in the arse to clean up (thanks to woodworm in the garage).

Ever since plans with the leather family fell through, we seemed to face one stumbling block after another. I had an offer on my house, but the sale of a new place we liked fell through. So, we set our sights as far as Eastbourne, and found a lovely house which was on a good, regular bus route to Brighton; an end-of-terrace property and 100 yards from the beach, an exceptionally good location. But the paperwork for the new house would take months to arrange, so we had to rent elsewhere in the meantime.

My two pussies, Flossie and George (poor Dottie had died a few months before), were not too sure where they were in this rented place. They had been used to a huge garden to roam around in my old house on the other side of Saltdean. One early morning I was up early and realised my favourite pussy George – I should not have a favourite, I know – was not around. I called and searched for him everywhere, panic-stricken, before I found him under the hedge by the front garden gate, dead and stiff. I wailed as I carried him inside to Angelo, and he too wept at the sight of our favourite pussy in my arms.

Neither of us knew what to do with a dead animal. After I had calmed down, I decided to bury him in the garden. I'm not sure it was permitted to bury an animal on rented property. Oh well.

"I'm buying a rosemary bush to place as his headstone," I declared, through sobs.

Angelo shot me a quizzical look.

"It represents remembrance," I continued tearfully, "it is believed to strengthen the memory, and I will never forget George".

I still feel a pang in my chest whenever I see a chunky black cat in the street. I call out George's name to them, but they never look back.

I was trying to stay positive about our move, but it seemed there were more hurdles in our way. The bathroom in Eastbourne was ghastly and had to be gutted, so we called in a favour with an old mate of mine, Rachel. Once an actress, she was now an interior designer, and so had a crew of workmen on hand to help. Her gang of builders drew up plans to alter the house to our requirements, but there was no chance of a quick move. There was a lot more work, expense, and planning permission from the surveyor to finish the house than we expected, and our already small resources were running out fast. New concrete wall supports, new steel beams, new flooring. What a project we had taken on, more like *Grand Designs* than a simple facelift for a Victorian terrace.

Christmas Day 2011 was strange. We decided to take boxes of belongings over to the new house, even though there was hardly a floor to walk on downstairs. It was also a particularly freezing December day, and the house didn't have any heating. But we didn't care, we just wanted to be there. I thought that if we settled into the house quickly, we could start more global research into our business. The reason for buying this property with no mortgage was to release funds for our business to move forward, after all. It seemed so ironic that it was now the main thing holding us back.

My last place was a beautiful, happy house, and it was Angelo's first UK home. I would never have moved if we weren't serious about creating a life together. So, there we were on this festive day, wandering around a half-finished, completely empty shell of a property, trying to imagine where to place the furniture. All we needed were walls to be finished and a floor to walk on. Not much really.

Early in 2012 we eventually moved over to Eastbourne and settled in. The builders had done a terrific job – the open space downstairs, once the dividing wall was secure, was roomy and light. Even Flossie, our one remaining cat, seemed to like the place. I chose the name Flossie some time back when I was reading a Minette Walters book. In the book, a prostitute called Flossie was brutally murdered with a hairbrush. Do not ask how it was used, it was a ghastly tale, but I loved the name.

First on our agenda was turning the spare bedroom into an office space for Angelo where he could sketch his designs. We bought drawing boards, a new computer, shelves to house folders upon folders of documents from our research days into 'how to set up your new business', stationery, you name it – an endless list of supplies.

It took over a year, all told, to move everything into Eastbourne. The entire moving process had been incredibly stressful and unsettling; it had taken a toll on us both. We had, however, made a beautiful home for ourselves, so I assumed everything would be okay again.

In our well-equipped and completed office upstairs at home, Angelo continued, when possible, to search for any kind of link into the leather fashion trade. He was not giving up on finding a way to use his elegant designs. We seemed to be making little headway, but he never stopped looking for an in.

We were still a happy couple, I believed, in those days. A fly on the wall watching us cuddle up on the sofa to watch television in the evenings would certainly think so. But, in a far corner of my mind, I could sense something was building up inside Angelo. I thought perhaps he was fed up with his long commute to work, which ate into his sketching time, or maybe it was the frustration of trying various avenues to jump-start our business together and not getting far.

CHAPTER TWENTY-ONE

Angelo was chattering more than usual. I hadn't seen him so uplifted in a long time. He had just arrived back from a leather fair in Alicante, and he was enthusiastically telling me all about a young Spanish guy he had met there, with whom he seemed to hit it off right away.

His name was Armando, he spoke English perfectly, and had shown a great interest in Angelo's ideas. Angelo had decided on another segue into the fashion industry, designing men's footwear, and as luck would have it, Armando was already working for a company manufacturing top-rate leather shoes. He wanted to move up the leather shoe trade ladder and be more active on the creative side in the same industry. So, it seemed like a good omen that they met. Plus, 'Angelo and Armando' would sound good on a letter heading. It looked promising.

Armando was helpful and friendly, and he realised that if he wanted to move up in this world, he needed a contact like Angelo to partner with. He was a brilliant contact for us to have, too, and it seemed like there was every possibility they could work hand in glove. With Angelo designing in England, and Armando finding factories to produce the first prototypes in Spain, production could begin quickly. It sounded ideal.

At the beginning, Angelo and Armando talked on the phone almost constantly, discussing possibilities to get something off the ground between them. Armando approached several factories to see if there was a way to make a deal. But the research in Spain was slow, and I could see that Angelo was getting frustrated that the process of trying to start up a business in another country was taking so long.

In a cruel twist of fate, in 2012 the economy in Spain began to flounder, then everything started to crash. Businesses were going down left, right, and centre, and the cost of living rose dramatically across the country. The outcome of our partnership in the Spanish leather market did not look so good – with such a huge financial disaster, Armando seemed to think that any factory would need large upfront payments to even consider creating small amounts of prototypes. All was looking glummer for us than before the trip to Alicante.

Dreams of a business together were disintegrating – it was a tough time. The stress of not getting far with the original plan was frustrating, to say the least. My career as an actor had brought with it many challenges, rejections, and disappointments over the years, so I was well used to the ups and downs of working life by now. But this wasn't the case for Angelo – he had nothing to gauge this experience on.

To make matters worse, Angelo was still travelling to and from work in Brighton on the bus. It was a tedious journey of about 45 minutes at best, but on cold and wet wintry days, when more people used the service, it took an hour for him to get home to Eastbourne. This certainly didn't aid productivity or creative inspiration. I knew he sometimes passed the time reading scriptures and sections of the Koran on his phone; perhaps he was seeking spiritual inspiration.

It was already almost two years since that wonderful time in Istanbul with the leather family, and we hadn't progressed any further in our plans. In fact, developing a business had only gone as far as the starting line. I had put my acting life on hold since our idea of working together had shown a glimmer of becoming a reality. It wasn't that I was really missing performing, but I knew our plan should have taken us further by now. Although that's not to say that I ever felt resentful – I had had huge successes over many years; I had quite a glittering career to look back on, in fact. It's just that I wanted the same glittering future with my partner. His designs were stunning, even to a layman like me, and it was totally frustrating to see they were not yet in production. But despite the stresses and setbacks in our work life, I felt our relationship was still strong – I was never given a reason to think otherwise.

On several occasions I tried to push Angelo to contact the Spaniard more often, thinking he should try more ways to persuade Armando to search for other options. Angelo, I feared, was not encouraging or pushing him enough and letting things slide by. I wanted him to contact Alicante almost daily. But after a day's work and a bus journey back home, he was not that enthusiastic about picking up the phone. Understandable, I suppose. Maybe I was interfering too much, trying to nudge him further. But this was my business too, and I usually like things to be done yesterday.

One evening, when Angelo got home from work and I was starting to cook dinner, I tried to persuade him, in no uncertain terms, to keep tabs on Armando. I was urging him to phone Spain regularly for news. Otherwise, I thought, if contact was eased off, even for a couple of days, there was a possibility the Spaniard may completely lose interest.

Suddenly, and quite unexpectedly, Angelo exploded: "You phone him yourself! *You* keep the contact going if you are so interested!"

I was taken aback, too stunned to retaliate. Such an unusually forceful statement coming from my otherwise laid-back, easy-going, smiley partner was a complete shock. It was so out of character – he never raised his voice at all. Ever. He seemed taken by surprise that I had begun to challenge him at all, and I was equally surprised at his outburst. We never really rowed over anything. We bickered a little, like any other couple, maybe over what to have for dinner or what to watch on the television, but we never once shouted at each other.

I could see he was mulling over what was said. But from that moment on, we did not speak to each other about the outburst. I put it down to stress and exhaustion. He practically stopped mentioning Armando at all after that evening. The Spanish connection was left in abeyance, so to speak.

But still, Angelo did not give up on his dream. A few weeks later, he was on his way back to Algiers, to a trade fair in his homeland. I believed visiting his own country would be good for him – he could breathe in a little of his culture and speak his language again for a while, and perhaps he may return refreshed and inspired, with new ideas of how we could progress.

Angelo did return with good contact links to a couple of businesses, but they were nothing whatsoever to do with fashion or his design ideas. One contact was with a cosmetics company, and he thought maybe he could be their representative or 'sole trader' in this country. As he was a dual citizen of Algeria and the UK, travelling back and forth to negotiate deals would be easy, he said.

It was not what we had envisaged doing when we originally decided to go into business together, but he seemed to think it had potential, so he was willing to give it a try. And I went along with it. Not a lot of choice, really. A new plan was better than no plan at all, I told myself.

He did seem refreshed from the trip, and more positive about this new venture. But things changed after he got back to Eastbourne. He returned from his day job one evening and announced that he wanted to start praying again. This statement came completely out of the blue. He said he had been thinking about his religion a lot, and he appeared to be a little nervous telling me this news.

Maybe mixing with his countrymen had triggered a yearning for his religion; maybe seeing mosques in the capital had rekindled his interest in Islam. I have no idea. I never asked him. We never really discussed his religion in any depth.

I must be honest when I explain that the feeling that came over me as I heard these words was as if someone was walking on my grave. Until this point, which was coming up to seven years since our civil partnership, I had learned comparatively little of Islam at all, primarily because Angelo never mentioned it. I was not against any part of the religion; I was just ignorant of it. But I knew that, like Christianity too, I suppose, it did not have a good history with the gay community, to put it lightly.

I had no idea what this return to faith meant for us. Would it make a difference to our lives as a gay couple? It was powerful news for me to take in, and I was suspicious as to why religion was suddenly being discussed for the first time in our relationship, in such a casual manner. Surely, he must have realised this would affect me directly.

Stupidly, I never asked Angelo how this announcement would affect me, or our relationship. I said shockingly little, to be honest. I wasn't sure of a response that was suitable.

I fear the unknown, it's always scared me. Bare facts laid out before me I can cope with well. The terrible, life-changing sequence of events brought on by Robert's illness and his untimely death, for instance, I had to accept. I knew what the outcome was going to be. This evening's announcement may not have been a terminal one, but the shock and uncertainty of it totally unnerved me.

I'm sure I looked slightly bewildered as Angelo told me his plans. But I loved this man, and I wanted him to be happy, so of course I told him I supported his decision.
"When do you intend to visit the local mosque?" I asked casually, later that evening over dinner.
"I'll go this coming Friday," he replied. He seemed to relax a bit at my acceptance.
"But you don't know where it is in this town, do you? Have you ever seen it?" I asked inquisitively.
He realised he didn't.
"I'll drive you there," I said with a smile. "I pass it often on the way to the supermarket." I wanted him to see that I was enabling him, in a way, to start his religious comeback. At least I understood how important Friday prayers were in the Islamic calendar.

Angelo explained that it was necessary for Muslims to complete five daily prayers: *Fajr* at dawn, *Dhuhr* at midday, *Asr* in the afternoon, *Magrib* at sunset, and *Isha* at night. I, again, wondered if and how this would disrupt our home life. I didn't know what the prayers sounded like or how long they lasted. Could I stay in the house during, or did he expect complete privacy at home? I had no idea. But, to show my solidarity, I visited a local shop in Eastbourne where I bought a small prayer mat. It was not particularly stylish or luxurious, but it was simply a token of my support.

So, Angelo began his daily prayers in our office room upstairs, and on Fridays, when he wasn't working in Brighton, I drove him over to the local mosque. For our relationship to work, it seemed an important thing for me to do, and I wanted to be a part of his new routine.

My only exposure to prayer was from my own Christian upbringing in the local church. As a child growing up in a small town in the late 50s and early 60s, I was ignorant of any religions other than Christianity. I knew there were Methodists, Roman Catholics, and Presbyterians locally, but they were simply different sections of the same religion. Words like Muslim, Islam, Hindu, Buddhist, Jewish, to my knowledge, were never explained or mentioned in regular day school, nor in Sunday school lessons. Clearly, I had a very closeted childhood, in more ways than one.

As a choirboy, I knew all the popular hymns and psalms because I learned the words by rote from hearing them so often. I now know that this was the same process for Muslim kids who can learn and recite the Koran, by heart, when they are very young. I was unaware whether my partner learned this way. He never mentioned it, and, once again, I never asked him.

Perhaps it was a mistake, in retrospect, that I never asked questions about his religion early on in our relationship. The only thing I did know was that his dad went to the mosque in his hometown every day, which seemed perfectly natural to me. But when Angelo was a rebellious teenager, to my knowledge, he eased off attending. That was the extent of my knowledge. Was it my fault, therefore, that he never spoke of Islam in the early days, because I had shown little interest in it? Was I to blame, in some way?

I knew that he was having a hard time with the constant setbacks to our business and his dream of being a designer. I had no definite proof of any of this, but my theory was that he was looking for an answer from Allah as to why his business ideas kept failing. After all, we often use the expression 'God help me' when something goes wrong in our lives. I guessed he was taking this expression more literally.

Maybe he thought not practising his religion was holding him back from being successful. Maybe he thought he was being held back because of his gay lifestyle. Maybe he thought he was being punished for loving and living with a man.

So many maybes.

CHAPTER TWENTY-TWO

The first proper Christmas in our new house was such an exciting time. As usual, I was ticking off my festive checklist: sending cards, buying gifts for friends. We decorated the house together – it wasn't a lesser Christmas because Angelo was a practising Muslim again. He always relished the festive period and all that goes with it. In fact, it was his yearly duty at work to mount the seasonal displays in the boutique shop windows. He was brilliant at it and the results were always spectacular. One year, when we lived in Saltdean, he spent hours putting together a display using piles of dried leaves, twigs, and branches from our garden, garnishing it with twinkling lights and glass baubles. The brothers who owned the business were always delighted with his artistic flair and eye-catching result; it really brought in the customers.

We had been asked to join our dear friends, Sophie and Nic Colicos – who lived a little distance away in Bexhill – for a festive Christmas meal. Sophie and I had worked together on several theatre productions over the years, so I knew her very well. She's a huge West End star now – a triumph in *Wicked* – as well as an amazing cook and a wonderful friend. I felt like a member of her family as her mum and dad, Audrey and Michael, often included me in their family celebrations.

"You realise our friends don't know of your decision to return to your faith yet," I said to him gently, as we were putting up our decorations, a couple of weeks before our planned festivities. "Wouldn't it be a good idea to let them know well before we visit them at Christmas?"
"Of course," he said. "I guess I had better mention to Sophie about me not eating meat these days, other than halal."
I had been shocked that halal meat in Eastbourne, in those days, was not easy to find. There was only one supermarket, Asda, that had an extremely limited supply, but no other supermarket chains in the town had any at all. I thought it odd

that all local supermarkets there had so little or no halal meat when the Muslim population in Eastbourne was huge.

"And I must also ask them about me praying in their house," Angelo added. "Do you think they will mind?" He seemed anxious.

"They're such lovely friends, I'm sure it will all be fine. You know what good people they are," I said reassuringly.

He nodded.

Sophie and Nic were terrific to honour Angelo's wishes, and they embraced his needs beautifully. Sophie cooked delicious fish for him while the rest of us ate a more traditional Christmas dinner. They were simply amazing and found a lovely quiet place for him to pray, alone, during the day. To them, he was a mate, and they respected his thoughts and his religion perfectly.

I had imagined my friends might have detected a change in him, in his mood or demeanour, when we arrived at their house that day, seeing as he was making so many changes within himself. But unless he arrived with two heads or a limb missing, they would, of course, see no change in him whatsoever. Why would they?

When others learned of Angelo's faith revival no one ever asked what this meant for our relationship, or if there was any conflict between us, what with me being, technically, a Christian man. Angelo was made to feel as comfortable and at ease with our other friends as he was with Sophie and Nic. His bosses, the wonderful Jewish brothers who owned the boutique, were wonderfully accepting, too. They made sure he had a private area to pray and went out of their way to make him feel comfortable at work.

At home, I was getting used to the prayer times and had no problem finding halal meat to eat. The imam of the local mosque was also a butcher, so I would wander down to his shop on many occasions and talk to this nice, friendly man about his tasty meat supplies. Mind you, I was missing the smell of bacon cooking, and I believed Angelo was too, to be honest.

**

We entered the new year in the same routine as the last: Angelo was working while I kept house. In the evenings, I'd pick him up from the town centre bus stop or drive over to Brighton to make his journey home quicker. I was trying my best to maintain our happy life together, but this more devout way of living had its complications, and I can't say it wasn't affecting me. I had begun to feel that I was treading very carefully with him. If we wanted to go shopping together or plan anything on his days off, it had to be on his schedule, according to the times of the prayers. "Let's go there earlier," he would say, or, "let's go there after prayers," and so on. It definitely hindered any chance of spontaneity, and Angelo had been such a spontaneous person; it was one of the things I loved about him. The prayer times were difficult for me to remember, too, as they followed the lunar calendar, and so changed depending on the time of year and the length of the days. It was a different way of living for him too, but it was his decision, so it was I who was adjusting to it more than he.

I had no idea if his family kept tabs on visits to the mosque when he first came to live with me in our Saltdean home, nor was I aware if they ever asked if he was following his faith generally when in England. Maybe they thought he was praying in the usual manner. Did they know that he had changed his daily routines by praying at home and visiting the mosque now each Friday?

Despite the changes in our life together, I still felt loved as spring approached in 2013. That Valentine's Day, I received the most beautifully written card and a stunningly wrapped gift. Angelo's presents were always selected carefully for each occasion, and his immaculate presentation was indicative of his creative talent. I had been so worried that his newfound faith would detrimentally affect our relationship, but his beautiful token truly put my mind at ease.

Yet, just days later, things began to change.

Being that we had been together for close to a decade and given that neither of us was the young stud we once may have been, our relationship was not a regularly rampant sexual one. Yet we had always been loving and affectionate with one another. But, as if out of nowhere, Angelo seemed to feel uncomfortable sleeping with me in our bedroom. He avoided even brushing up against me in bed, and he resigned himself to the far edge of the mattress so that he was out of my arms' reach. I was totally horrified. Truthfully, I felt ghastly. It was as though I repulsed him. I told myself that we had just passed the honeymoon phase, that was all. I ignored the phrase 'seven-year itch' that crept into my thoughts.

I loved sleeping next to Angelo, not just for sexual reasons, but for the warmth and comfort of my lover's body near me, plus the night-time chats we usually had about the events of the day. This was a big change to deal with. Part of me was angry after years of there being no issues in that department, but I was trying hard to keep him happy. So, to make living together non-confrontational, and to please him, I went along with the plan that he would start to sleep in our office. We had a sofa-bed in there already for guests who came to stay, and he wouldn't have to leave the room to pray.

The thing was, he wasn't just growing distant in the bedroom, I was also beginning to miss the cosy evenings when we would cuddle up on the sofa in front of the telly, with Flossie sitting nearby. We rarely even did this anymore. For the last seven years together, our home had been filled with love and warmth. Now I was beginning to feel it change; it was growing cold.

CHAPTER TWENTY-THREE

One evening after Angelo returned from work, he went to pray upstairs while I cooked us dinner, like any other day. I could tell he wasn't in the best frame of mind, however. It had been a dull, cold day in February, and he had just spent an hour on a crowded bus, so I thought this was understandable. But when he came back downstairs, he barely ate a mouthful of his dinner; he just pushed the food around his plate, which was disconcerting as it was one of his favourite dishes – fried fish with spinach and sauteed potatoes.

It was obvious that something was wrong. He was clearly on edge. He barely spoke – in fact, he had hardly said two words since he got through the door, and his sullen expression remained unchanged. I almost asked if I had done something to offend him, but he appeared not to be open to much of a discussion. So, we sat in unusually awkward silence.

The atmosphere in our house was unsettling and I couldn't understand why. Cooking and eating together were always our favourite moments to share with each other. Angelo could not seem to relax, and as I cleared away the dinner things, my stomach was churning in anticipation that something was about to happen.

Sure enough, all of a sudden, he blurted out: "Can we go out for a walk?"
I was perplexed and even more unnerved by his request. A perfectly reasonable thing to ask on a long summer evening, especially as we were living so near the beach. But it was after dark in mid-February, which meant it was positively Baltic outside.
"Go out right now, you mean?" I asked, completely flummoxed. He didn't respond. There had been a note of desperation in his voice, so I decided not to argue with him.

"Okay then," I said, as breezily as I could manage. "We'd better put on some warm coats, it'll be cold out there."
We both donned our outdoor clothes in uncomfortable silence. The beach by our home was less than a hundred yards away. Alongside the stretch of pebbles was a promenade that led towards a pier. We awkwardly, and briefly, discussed the weather, as though we were complete strangers, but as I had no idea why we were out walking on this freezing February evening I said extraordinarily little else.

Aside from the odd dog walker we passed on the beach path, we were completely alone, walking against the wind. Bizarrely, when we got to the pier, we turned around in unison to walk the same route back, still without saying a word to each other. This miserable walk Angelo had so desperately requested was not producing anything other than frozen faces. Clearly, it had made no difference to his attitude, the existence of which continued to perplex me as he was never moody. His trademark grin seemed like a distant memory.

I took off my outdoor coat as soon as we were through the front door. I was preparing to settle down and thaw out, but within seconds of stepping inside, he broke his streak of silence.
"Can we go for a drive? I need to go out again."
I gawped at him in consternation.
"What, now? We've just been out…"
"I want to go out somewhere," he reiterated firmly. "I just don't want to stay in."
I don't know why I didn't challenge him right there and then about this odd behaviour. I just agreed to drive, all around areas of Eastbourne I had never seen before, and never want to see again.

I kept driving to please him, and once more tried talking pleasantries about the weather. I had thought he would want to find a place to stop, to maybe have a drink somewhere and talk. I was sure that he wanted to say something important. But he was practically mute. Still, I didn't question him at all. I was frankly scared to delve deeper into the problem. Mostly, I was concerned about his state of mind. He was behaving as I had never seen him do so before. Maybe something was radically wrong. Surely if he were ill or unwell he would tell me immediately and I could help him – God knows I'm a good carer. But that evening, when we returned home, he went straight up the stairs to bed without another word, although I could see he was far from tired.

I did not know what to say or do to help, so, dumbfounded, I followed him upstairs, parting ways at our separate bedrooms, as he went to sleep in what we had hoped would be his office. I felt physically sick as I got ready for bed; I tried to sleep but my mind simply would not let me rest. I replayed the evening's misadventure over and over again. Our happy life together seemed to be floundering, and I had no idea how to fix it.

The next morning, I was up early (in truth, I barely slept a wink). I presumed that Angelo was going to work after breakfast – he usually made his way to the bus stop at the end of our road to get the bus into Brighton – so I made breakfast and coffee, and sat in the living room waiting to talk to him. I presumed he would want to say something about last night's weird episode.

He came downstairs, fetched himself a coffee, and sat on the sofa, without so much as a 'good morning'.
Then he looked over at me, stone-faced, and out of nowhere said softly: "I feel I have to go from here now, and I am sorry".
His voice was wobbly. Not a long speech at all, just a matter-of-fact announcement. My now sweaty palms were losing grip of the coffee mug I was grasping on to for dear life.
"What? What are you talking about?" I asked gently, trying – failing – to remain calm. "Where are you going?"
I repeated this several times, to no response.
Eventually, he mustered a reply: "I must leave here. It's not right that I am living here with you, and I must go."
So simple a statement; direct and final. He wouldn't look at me, he just stared ahead, unmoving, just as I was frozen with shock. This was clearly what had been on his mind on our strange evening walkabout last night. I suspected something epic was evolving in our lives. I had no idea it would be this.

"What are you saying?" I asked repeatedly, like a cracked record. I was desperate for some clarity, but there was no answer. His whole demeanour was so radically different from the man I knew. My smiley person had morphed into a cruel, cold, unfeeling stranger.

I knew it must be his faith that was dividing us. I understood it was against the Islamic laws to have sex and live with a man, but the fact that it was haram had never, ever been an issue between us before. Just as Christian beliefs had never impacted us. Surely this was something that he might have thought about well before we had a civil partnership ceremony, seven years ago. Why was this happening now?

I felt as though a physical hole had appeared in the base of my stomach. The only other time I remember having such a hideous feeling was the day I learned my Robert would die. It was back with a vengeance. Total loneliness. Total emptiness.

It was so quick a change for me to process. I never expected his religion would take him away from me like this. Of course, there had been a build-up of change in him from the time he started to pray at home. Then the progressive move to not sleeping with me in the same bed or even in the same room. But, surely, we could live together as loving friends in the same house. He could still follow his faith at the same time; after all, we had been doing this for the last three months.

I knew he could see that I was visibly astounded by his announcement. I was trying to be an adult about this devastating news, but on the inside, I was absolutely furious. Seething. But I didn't raise my voice at him, which surprised me at the time. Perhaps if I had yelled, I may have gotten more of a response, rather than this frigid silence. I should have gone over to him to shake his shoulders and demand a more believable answer.

But I didn't. I was frozen to the chair.

There was no discussion, no pleading. This was a fait accompli.

"Where are you going to stay if you're leaving now?" I asked flatly.

"I might stay over with a friend for a few nights," he muttered.

It was too ridiculous to comprehend he was leaving on the spur of the moment – we had lived together with no issues for years, for goodness' sake. This was insane. Or was I insane?

If only he could tell me something like: "I have fallen in love with another guy from up the road and I'm going to be with him". I would be shocked and angry about an affair, but it would somehow feel like a more rational scenario. At least I would have something, or someone, to rail against. But, of course, there was no one behind the scenes to run away with. It was simply his religion he was returning to. Running to – fast, it seemed.

I searched his once kind face for an answer. He looked dreadful. The eyes that had looked at me with love for years were sunken and brimming with tears; his gleaming smile was concealed by pursed lips. He said he was going upstairs to pack a case, still refusing to look me in the eye. I, by now, was in a kind of catatonic state, sitting motionless in the armchair. Nothing was making sense.

This breakfast-time episode, which radically altered my life, was at most 20 minutes long. After only a few minutes more, Angelo reappeared downstairs with a suitcase in tow. I was standing in the hallway waiting for him, stunned and confused, but somehow not tearful in the slightest. I have no idea how, or why, I didn't cry. I felt helpless to even grab his suitcase to stop him from going. Short-term partnerships may run their course when it's time to move on, but we were in a different league, or so I had thought.

I stood behind him in the hallway as he opened our front door and trundled his wheelie suitcase over the path and down to the bus stop. I remained in the empty hall, looking at the back of the closed front door for a few moments, rigid in fright.

In the recesses of my mind, I knew I had had a niggling feeling that Angelo's religion would, in some way, be reintroduced. I had no idea how or exactly when. But in that moment, standing frozen in the doorway, I was suddenly reminded of an event that happened several years before my partner had been recalled to his faith.

During my theatre time touring the country with various productions over the years, I worked in the Derby Theatre a couple of times. There I had a great landlord called John, who became a dear friend. At the time, he had a terrific British-Pakistani boyfriend who was years younger than he (the age difference between them was about the same as my relationship). They were a great couple; I saw them together regularly and they were perfectly happy. They were clearly devoted to each other over the several years I knew them. But John told me, on more than one occasion, that he was convinced his young man would leave him one day because of his religion. He believed that he would be persuaded to marry a Muslim girl.

I never believed that would ever happen, it seemed impossible to comprehend that he would ever contemplate being persuaded into marrying any girl. John, however, said he was convinced that it would change between them one day and he was prepared for it, should it happen. Indeed, it did.

John's young partner had several girls presented to him by his family who lived locally, but he rejected them, claiming he wasn't ready for marriage. But more and more girls were presented to him, and eventually, he caved. He chose one and married her. Whether his decision was brought about by his parents' religious beliefs, his own, societal pressures, or a combination of the three, I don't know. But I do know that everything changed for John that day.

All I could think to do was call Lesley.
"Hello darling," I blurted out, and then I became silent.
"What's up? You sound weird."
"He's gone."

"What are you talking about?"

I told her, briefly, what had happened. She too was speechless at the news.

"I'll call him now to see if he will talk to me."

"He's gone to the Brighton bus stop already."

"I'll call him and call you back."

I waited for a moment or two before the phone rang in my hand.

"He was at the bus stop with his suitcase, waiting for the bus. He was crying a lot and was not very coherent at all as he spoke to me."

The image of him weeping in the street 100 yards from our house was utterly devastating. If he really wanted to be away from me, surely he should be in a happier state of mind, not in fits of tears.

"He believes he can't practise his religion as he now feels he should, whilst living with a man," Lesley explained.

She also gleaned from him, in between his sobs, that he didn't want to hurt me.

"Didn't want to hurt me," I spat, "bit late for that, isn't it?"

"You shouldn't be alone, darling," Lesley said gently.

She suggested that I go visit a friend as soon as possible. Thankfully, I had already arranged to visit Tony and Christine in Saltdean that day, so even though the floodgates had now opened, and I was completely hysterical, I decided to drive over. I needed to see friendly faces who knew us both well. They had entertained us on so many occasions, as an equally happy couple.

I'm sure they weren't expecting me to arrive in such a state. They both tried to console me with affirmations like, "He'll change his mind", and "This is only a blip". But their words were of little comfort when my gut screamed the opposite. Sure enough, the hours passed and there was no sign of Angelo, proving this was much more than just a bump in the road. I told my nearest and dearest friends my news. Each time I called them it was difficult to get the words out.

At some point, Angelo called me. It could have been one day or several after his exodus – I wasn't sure how long he had been away by then; I had no concept of time. He was staying with one of his girlfriends from work, sleeping on her sofa. He told me several times about how very sorry he was that this had happened. I appeared to be developing mental issues due to the suddenness of this split – I couldn't fully register the conversation, so I could say very little in response. But I do remember these words: "In the future, you will see this is the best thing for me to do for my religion, and it will turn out to be the best thing to happen to you, too".

I yelled back at him some obscenity because it seemed like a stupid, heartless statement to make to me right then, especially as I was clearly completely unhinged at that time.

"Why was it not possible to be living at the same address as friends and for you to still follow your religion?" I asked him, several times. There was a brief pause. Then he spoke calmly, almost as though he had rehearsed what he wanted to say, or was reading from a page in front of him.

"I couldn't stay in the house," he replied, quietly. "We simply cannot jump from living together in a house as civil partners to becoming just housemates in the same place."

Who on earth had impressed these rules and regulations on him, I wondered? How did this happen to us in such a short space of time? Just a few days ago, on Valentine's Day, I had felt so loved. Now I felt totally unwanted, and useless.

Nothing made sense. I was going insane trying to understand it all. I still haven't fully figured it out.

CHAPTER TWENTY-FOUR

For more than a year or so I had been practising Pilates with an instructor in Eastbourne, Jane Cramer. Jane was a lovely lady, and it had been a fun way to keep fit, but in the weeks after Angelo left, it became more than that. It became vital for my health. Jane started to help me to unwind, physically – I was practically tied up in knots – and encouraged me to at least try and relax in our sessions. There were times with her when I wept as I let go of all the tension I had been harbouring. She expected it.

I told her my personal issues; she was a great listener and an expert instructor. She could physically see the difference in the way I stood and walked. She saw the stress in my body and heard its effect on my voice. As an actor, any tension affects the voice dramatically, and I was seriously tense, so my once strong, clear voice was now dull and flat. I knew that continuing the process of regular Pilates with her would not only help ease my tense body, but also certainly help to relax my mind.

What was happening in my private life was not going to be resolved quickly, but these sessions were taking the edge off, at least. At this moment in my life, I was so glad to have met Jane Cramer. I felt that I was in good hands.

Over the last couple of weeks at home, alone, the events leading up to my break-up had been playing on repeat in my head, like an omnibus of a terrible soap. But no matter how much I mulled it over, I simply could not make sense of it. Angelo was having some sort of religious epiphany, the introduction of which changed everything for me, and it seemed there was no going back. But I was not sure how to go forward.

Jane's studio was a car journey away from my house. As I finished my session one morning, I received a text from Angelo to say that he was on his way back to Eastbourne to see me. It was a complete shock. Perhaps he wanted to talk to me about our future – or lack of it – together, or perhaps he was just in need of more clothes.

I knew that this face-to-face moment had to arrive sooner rather than later, so I quickly drove home, parked up, and waited. When he arrived, having not seen him for three weeks, I couldn't believe what he looked like.

Angelo was handsome, and, as I have said many times before, he was blessed with a radiant smile which rarely left his face. But today, he looked like someone else entirely – I hardly recognised him. His face was ashen and unshaven; his eyes dark and hollow, like he was possessed. Haunted, I would say. As though he had been locked up in a faraway prison and not seen much light of day. He looked ill, and decidedly unhappy.

The stress of the last few weeks had obviously hit him badly. Considering what I was going through, I thought I looked rather a lot better than he did, which gave me solace. Compared to him, I was sure I appeared to be coping better on the surface, but I wished he could look inside my head to see the mangled ball of emotional wool that filled it.

I welcomed him into the house – no hugs from either of us, just general, stilted politeness. He seemed pleased to be back. Almost immediately, he asked if he could go to bed and sleep, if I didn't mind. Such an odd thing to ask of your ex-partner after not seeing each other for three weeks, but he was visibly weak from lack of sleep and seemed ready to keel over with exhaustion. So, I agreed he must go to bed for a rest. He was very grateful.

I presumed he might want to go to the office bedroom to sleep as before, but no, he chose to climb into the big, comfortable bed we had shared for years. Then, and I cannot believe I did this, I tucked him in. He just looked so pathetic and ill.

Angelo slept there for quite some time. I stayed, watching him sleep for a little while, trying to understand the events that had led to this moment as I looked down at him. An hour or so later, he woke and came downstairs, and I gave him something to eat and drink in the living room. Then we began to chat. What a weird situation – it was almost as though I was about to interview him, but I wasn't sure of the right questions to ask.

I gathered that he needed belongings to take away, given that he had had a huge wardrobe yet had only taken one hastily packed suitcase with him weeks before. And he certainly needed a good shave. He had been sleeping rather rough on sofas at various girlfriends' homes recently and it showed.

Was it permissible for a single Muslim man to stay overnight with an unmarried girlfriend, even if he was sleeping on the sofa? Was it not forbidden to do so, especially if she was unaccompanied? Perhaps there was an exemption if the female was giving shelter to someone in distress? Who knows. I was just glad he had those women to help him.

This strange day meeting up, after such an absence, was the time to work out a plan for if we were irrevocably splitting up. A part of me still hoped that we could live together as housemates, especially as we were clearly good friends. But it was agreed, there and then, that he would return very soon to Eastbourne for a few weeks to complete our break-up arrangements. We needed time, to sort out the relationship status, and all our possessions, so we decided it was best for him to stay in the house and sleep in the office bedroom. It was simply practical.

We needed to officially separate our lives in an orderly, sensible fashion. It was going to be a hideous process. We were civil partners after all, and just like any other divorcing couple, we had joint bank accounts, and our names were on so many official documents – council tax, business plans, and so on. It was as tedious as it sounds.

Of course, he needed a new address to show employers, banks, and prospective landlords, so he needed to start looking for a place to live. I made it clear it would be best if he could leave our address by the beginning of the next fiscal year in a few weeks' time.

Who would ever imagine that we would be having a conversation about divorce after facing such a struggle to be together in the first place?

To give Angelo his due, one of the first things he insisted I do was completely change my will and leave nothing for him. I did, after all, own the house we were living in. He insisted, honourably, that he wanted nothing from me, and when he returned for the last month, that was the first thing I did. I hated doing it. He had become my entire world – officially exempting him from my will made the end of it so final.

Surprisingly, you might think, the last few weeks we spent together in Eastbourne weren't awkward for either of us. I showed no animosity towards him or his religious life choice; I wasn't resentful of him, although I believed there had been times when I really had just cause to be.

Obviously, the business that we had been planning for the last several years was scrapped. The dream of working together had gone up in smoke. So much time and energy had gone into it, visiting seminars and trade workshops. We had spent an enormous amount of money too, equipping our office and visiting trade fairs in Turkey, Spain, and Algeria. For nothing.

No use crying over spilt milk, I tried to tell myself, but it was heartbreaking dismantling our neat office in the spare bedroom, disposing of filing cabinets, endless files, and boxes. Small things that had, at one time, symbolised our hope for the kind of future we could build together. Things that once seemed so vitally important, cast aside like rubbish.

Undoing our relationship this way was horrendous. It was hard trying to be strong for my own preservation during this period. But I must move forward, I thought, even if I felt like an empty shell of myself.

I never wanted it to be over. I always presumed that this relationship was for the long haul. The last time I became a single man was because Robert died so tragically. It was the most horrendous time to live through. This was different, of course, but it was the death of a relationship – it certainly felt like a form of bereavement.

I was determined to try and survive this dreadful episode in my life, somehow. What a task ahead of me, though.

CHAPTER TWENTY-FIVE

I began to think I was either going mad or having a nervous breakdown. This entire episode of my life was so totally unexpected and unbelievable that I had no measure of whether or not I was reacting normally. I was living in a town where I knew very few people and believed I had no function or purpose in life. Sleep was non-existent; I wept for most of the night instead. I realised it was going to take a lot more than Pilates to stop my mind from working overtime at night. My friends had been amazingly supportive, but, seeing as I was losing my marbles, I clearly needed something more.

My local doctor in Eastbourne happened to be a Muslim man. I visited him again as soon as I was able. I was in a jabbering state as I nervously explained that my male Muslim partner of many years was leaving me. Explaining the religious aspect of my marital split to this man of the very same religion was extraordinarily awkward. I found it difficult to even look him in the face in case he was not understanding of my situation. Would he take pity on me? Would he approve of my visit at all?

He could see I was visibly shaken as I asked him for medication to sleep. He was incredibly sympathetic and kind; he seemed to understand my predicament and was completely non-judgemental, which was a blessing. He listened and avoided passing any kind of remark on the religious side of the split. As he calmly spoke to me, he used the expression "your personal upset" when he was referring to the reason I was in his surgery. This carefully chosen phrase was a relief to hear.

I imagine I must have appeared more than a little disturbed, especially as I was asking for sleeping pills to numb my mind. The doctor informed me – firmly, but still kindly – that he was not recommending medication because he thought I might do something silly and harm myself. But he wanted to help, so, within a remarkably short period of time, the caring doctor arranged for me to meet a local counsellor, named Valerie. Her office was a five-minute walk from my house and sessions were to begin at 2.00pm every Monday, after Angelo had finally vacated the house. I had no idea what to expect, but I knew I needed help from an impartial source.

All things considered, I coped rather well emotionally when Robert died, thanks to the amazing support from teams of medical people and close friends. But at that time, I had known he was HIV positive for more than a year. This was followed by a six-month period of watching his health fail as I nursed him at home to his untimely death. Those many months prepared me for the final blow. But that emotional trial I experienced all those years ago was completely different a chance to get used to the end of the relationship – it all happened too quickly to take in.

On the day of my first session with Valerie, I was nervous and arrived way too early, circling the block a couple of times before I walked through the doors of the reception area. It was a standard, National Health place. A bit cold, but Valerie greeted me warmly and said: "Let's go upstairs to a quiet room so we can talk".

We climbed the stairs to a room at the top of the building away from the world below. It was small, functional, and indeed quiet, with three office-style chairs placed around a small table. We chose a chair each and sat facing each other. Valerie placed a blank notebook on a smaller table beside her, preparing, I assumed, to jot down my innermost thoughts and troubles. Although, when the session began, I'm sure the poor woman must have thought that I was a bit thick – I could hardly speak much at all during my first session with her. I was tightly wound; I didn't know what I was supposed to say.

Actors have anxiety dreams when they're stressed about work, usually you're in a play waiting to go on stage and you realise with a jolt that you have no idea what your lines are, or what your role is in the production. Here, I had no idea of the production, the lines to say, how to articulate the character's emotions, or how the fuck I got the part in the first place.

I just sat there, staring straight ahead to avoid her gaze. But she was kind and patient as she waited for me to tell her something relevant about my agitated mental state. I knew she could only help or discuss my problems with me if I told her what they were, but it was as though my mouth just couldn't form the words. There were moments of almost complete silence as I clammed up, wringing my hands together. She did have some background knowledge from my doctor, so she knew why I was there in the first place, but she didn't pry.

I had been expecting Valerie to bombard me with questions so that I could begin to open up to her, but I soon realised that was not how it worked. Eventually, as each of these sessions with this charming lady unfolded, I started to unwind. I managed to tell her everything, bit by bit, that was causing me so much pain and confusion. She had endless patience as I slowly related what was going on in my head. She was an extraordinary listener. I'm surprised she was able to understand me at all – my words were jumbled, and I wept almost constantly. She too shed a gentle tear as my tale unfolded.

She was never judgemental. In fact, I felt she was on my side of the fence during our meetings. She liked me, I could tell, and I really began feeling more comfortable with this easy-going lady. She was like a favourite aunty.

It may sound strange, given that I spent most of the time in tears, but my Monday afternoons during that whole summer were incredibly special. I really looked forward to them. Sharing the burden of my turmoil with this total stranger was, slowly, giving me a new lease of life. I knew that when I left that little room, every week, I would feel just that tiny bit happier than before. It was a slow process, but I felt my spirits lift after each session with Aunty Valerie. She even made me laugh on the odd occasion, which was a miracle in itself. It was something in the week to look forward to. There was bugger all else to cheer me up.

I started to feel I could move forward. The wool was unravelling. I was beginning to breathe again.

After each session with Valerie, spilling my heart out, I walked home via the best Italian ice cream parlour in Eastbourne, near the seafront. There I'd buy a double scoop of something tasty and walk home along the beach and promenade whilst licking my favourite flavour. I began to find joy again, in those moments, strolling calmly on a sunny day, eating my ice cream.

The walk home was poignant. The route along the promenade to my front door was the same one Angelo and I took on that cold, miserable, February night. My sessions not only helped me to talk my way back into some sort of life, but they started to erase that awful promenade walk home, months earlier. From here on, there was little for me to fear walking that familiar path, apart from getting melted ice cream on my T-shirt.

I was still going through a bereavement; part of my life was slowly fading away and suddenly there was a huge void in its place. The only certain thing ahead was a future as a bewildered, single man living in the wrong town, but at least I was now facing it full on. And as time passed, my anger and confusion and hurt started to fade.

I had not been working as an actor for some time, having put my career on hold in the hopes of getting our own business off the ground. It had been a four-year break away from theatre work; a rather long hiatus. I missed it.

Then, out of the blue, things changed – an opportunity came my way. I was asked to attend a birthday party, miles away from my house in Eastbourne, in Wivelsfield. As I was not a great party lover, and never knew who to talk to first if I did go, my response would usually have been some form of, "No, thanks". In the recent past, I often used an excuse like, "So sorry we can't come to the party, Angelo won't be back from work in time". But this time I couldn't use that way out. I had to go.

To my surprise – relief – it turned out to be a rather fun night. And then, towards the end of the evening, the host, Janet Allen, who had worked with Robert years ago, came over to where I was sitting and asked me if I was interested in directing a play, a copy of which she was holding in her hand, waving at me.

"No, fuck off!" I exclaimed in mock horror.

She laughed. I had known her for years by this point.

"Now look, you cheeky so and so," she said, pretending to scold me. "I insist that you at least take it home with you and read it."

I rolled my eyes at her and smiled, promising I would take a look, although I had no real interest in playacting, directing, or performing in anything in those post-Angelo days. Even though I missed working, it still felt too soon to take on such a project – I didn't think my mind was equipped to cope with the chaos of live theatre quite yet.

So, the play – *Skirmishes*, by Catherine Hayes – lay on a table for a while, gathering dust, in my empty, lonely house. I tried to ignore it for as long as I could, until one day I felt compelled to read it. It was a story of old age and dementia, and it was both funny and tragic. I loved it. I had been out of the game for a while, and I had certainly never directed anything myself before, but as apprehensive as I was, I knew it could work well. Maybe. I should at least talk to Janet about it again, I thought to myself.

The play had a small cast of three women, which meant that the casting process wouldn't be a monumental task, at least.

"I'm sure we could find actresses to play the roles," I told Janet over a coffee, a couple of weeks after her party, "but how can we do a play without someone to produce it? We'd need a bit of cash to even hire the theatre space."

"We could all pull together to get it on its feet," Janet said confidently.

"Yes," I said, "I suppose we could".

I could tell she was eager to put on the show, and she really seemed to think I was best suited for the job. Indirectly, this meant that despite my initial reluctance, and without really applying for the job, I suddenly became both director and producer.

I felt a compelling urge to succeed in this theatre project, even though I was still reeling from the commotion of the last few months. It was a thrilling new adventure to be involved with, so I decided to dive in, mainly to occupy my mind and forget my loneliness.

The plan was to perform the play at the next Brighton Fringe Festival, which by then was months away the following year. I decided to try my hand at raising funds for the production. I discovered various crowdfunding campaigns on the internet which were a great way to get the production costs paid. Friends, I hoped, would help, and theatre-loving angels, too. I quickly prepared a campaign, producing a grainy video of myself explaining why the play needed to be performed, then set up the fundraising platform with photos of the three actresses and me, along with our biographies. I'd never ventured into this type of thing before, but I found myself enjoying it.

This new period in my life, arranging this production, triggered happy memories of my lately ignored, chosen acting career. I didn't think I would ever appear as an actor again. There's nothing like the smell of the grease-paint or the roar of a crowd, and it was so uplifting to be around fellow theatre people; as brilliant as Valerie was, this was truly the best therapy to help me through one of the most difficult times in my life.

Once armed with a little cash from the team of four, I bought and painted second-hand furniture from local charity shops. The small group and I found endless props and costumes bought the same way, very cheaply, with our collective piggy banks. The completed cast was comprised of three lovely professional actresses living in East Sussex: Janet Allen, who had found the play in the first place; Alexa Povah, one of my best friends, who

I'd worked with years before in repertory; and the lovely Cherith Mellor.

The money we raised from crowdfunding helped pay for some of the basic production costs. After hours upon hours of rehearsals, opening night at the Brighton Fringe was upon us. My directorial debut. I was shitting myself. I couldn't believe people had paid money to see something I had directed. Mad.

We thought we would barely make any money from the performances. For each of us, it was our first time performing at the Fringe, which is always a risky business. There were so many plays, events, and performances, and all that choice meant people could decide to go and see something better. Most productions would be lucky to get two, possibly three, consecutive performances. We were booked for the week's run.

The response far surpassed any of our expectations – we even ended up making enough to cover all our costs. But the money wasn't important. We were doing it simply for the joy and love of theatre. Considering I'd never directed, nor produced, a Fringe production before, it was a bloody successful night in my books.

As luck would have it, within three days of our Fringe production ending its run in Brighton, I received a phone call from the amazing choreographer, Stephen Mear, whilst I was driving along the seafront.
"Hello dear, have you retired?"
I chuckled at his enquiry. I assumed he asked this because he and other theatre people hadn't seen me around over the last few years. They must have wondered where on earth I'd been.
"Hi there," I said. "I've not done much theatre of late myself, but I've just directed my first play on the Fringe."
"Well..." he paused dramatically before he delivered the news, which was fitting, "we wanted to know if you were interested in returning to Chichester. There is a part you can play in a new production of *Amadeus* I'm staging this summer."
I nearly dropped the phone, which I should not have been using while driving, I know.

"Of course," I said, trying – failing – to remain calm. "Yes, I want to work with you again, I would be totally insane not to!"

I couldn't believe this stroke of long-awaited good fortune. Stephen's magic wand had delivered Dr Theatre to my rescue. A role had fallen right in my lap, completely out of the blue, at the very same theatre where I was appearing when I first met Angelo on the internet dating site all those years ago. A complete nine-year cycle from beginning to end.

**

Theatre work seemed to come my way again after being invited back to Chichester. There was a tour of an Ayckbourn play, then a short run in a London theatre musical. I had no idea why these jobs arrived just after one of the lowest times of my life. Perhaps the theatre gods were looking out for me.

As a result of the unorthodox breakdown of my relationship, I sold our house in Eastbourne. I began to hate the building we had chosen as our home together – there were too many memories for me to be living there alone. I moved back to Brighton within the year.

EPILOGUE

After the dramatic ending of the relationship with my partner, I began to question myself as to why I didn't know more about the Islamic religion and understand a little more as to why he ended our time together. All I knew basically when we first met was there were places called mosques where Muslims would go to pray. I knew there were several prayers said there each day, and that Friday was the most religious of days to attend and pray. Several times I had heard the call for prayers from the mosque when walking by, and realised I'd also witnessed it on television shows. That's about all I knew to be honest.

My knowledge of the rules, regulations, and etiquette of the Islamic religious festivals when we were living together was one of complete ignorance.

That was because the holiest Islamic festival of Ramadan was never celebrated in our home during our time together, so therefore there were no questions from me to ask what the festival was about. Now I fully understand how important this period is for all Muslim communities. I understand the Islamic calendar is based on the lunar cycle, unlike the more common European solar-based Gregorian calendar. All this and more I have learned. But why on earth didn't I ask questions, why didn't we discuss his religion fully so that I could appreciate and understand how important it was to him? Was I therefore to blame in some way?

Some months after the dust had settled, and I was living alone in my new house in Brighton, I heard there was going to be an open day at the local mosque that coming Sunday.

I was curious. It had been two years since Angelo had left. I'd learned basic facts about Islam and the lifestyle that went with it in the last few months of our relationship. I knew people prayed regularly, a few times a day, and, of course, I had driven Angelo to the mosque in Eastbourne for Friday prayers. I wanted to know more, and I'd also never been inside the building itself; I had no idea what it looked like behind the outer walls.

Perhaps I would find something inside that maybe I had been missing all my life. Perhaps I would finally understand the pull Angelo felt to return to his religion, just by being inside their holy place. Maybe then I could truly heal.

So, when Sunday came around, I decided to go.

I was surprised at the huge, friendly welcome from the volunteers standing on the street corner near the mosque, guiding people to the main door. It seemed there was a slow trickle of visitors all day, of all ages and backgrounds.

"Can you take your shoes off and place them on the shoe rack over there, please?" one of the helpers, an older man dressed in a robe asked as we arrived. "You can collect them later as you leave."

Everyone entering obliged.

"If all the visitors would like to go upstairs to the display room, you're invited to look around up there and ask questions, if you want," another, younger, volunteer said warmly, with a smile.

In said display room, there were screens showing videos that explained all sorts of religions, not just Islam. There was also an extensive array of information leaflets and literature, and copious amounts of deliciously fresh food. They had gone to a lot of trouble for people, like me, to understand the Islamic religion, and feel at home. Not that they were there to convert us visitors that day.

Visitors were invited to wander around at our leisure to see all the presentations and given an open invitation to ask the imams present any questions we had about Islam. The biggest surprise was that most of the Muslims I spoke with appeared to know more about Jesus than I did. I had no idea that there was a chapter in the Koran devoted to Mary, Jesus's mother, either. Imagine me, a Christian choirboy, knowing less about my religion than some of these people present.

The only question I could think to ask the imam was the very same one I had asked the butcher in Eastbourne all those months ago: "How do local Muslims buy their halal meat in this city? I rarely found a huge variety of choices in all the local supermarkets when I lived in Eastbourne." Pathetic question to ask, I realise. Maybe I should have asked the imam about his views on homosexuality and gay rights in Islam; maybe I should have told him my own personal story and how my entire life was altered due to loving a Muslim man.

But I had lived through the shock of the split with my partner, and, these days, I was feeling slightly better adjusted. Slightly. So, I thought, why argue my own case at this late stage? Besides, I could never win an argument with an imam on my own personal points of view of their religion.

So, I said nothing on that subject. Maybe I was wrong not to ask about an issue that affected my life so dramatically and abruptly. But that really wasn't the point of my visit. I came to the open day that Sunday simply because I was curious about Islam and wanted to see the inside of a mosque. I wanted to observe. There was no ulterior motive.

What I didn't know anything about months ago, and have discovered since writing this account, is that there are various gay Muslim groups. There are men and women who follow their faith but still have either a gay partner or balance their gay lifestyle with their religion. This has been a total revelation to me and something that was never explored or discussed with my partner. Would it have made any difference at all if we had chatted about such a subject? I have no idea. His mind was clearly made up to choose the faith above the relationship at all costs.

After I explored the vast displays of information in the room upstairs, I sat down and ate a hearty, spicy lamb meal, and sipped coffee while I chatted with other visitors. There was quite a diverse section of the local population attending this open day and it was a completely relaxing experience. Then the call for prayers announcement came over the speaker.

This was the one thing I wanted to avoid whilst I was inside this building. After all, it was this call to prayer within Angelo that triggered the end of our relationship, there's no denying it. Despite how well the day had started, and how welcoming everyone had been, at that moment I was not sure I wanted to be there anymore.

But then a soft-spoken young man approached me and said, kindly: "If you're at all interested in watching them during prayers, I can take you downstairs and show you where to sit".

I don't think he was singling me out, for any reason, and he wasn't pushing the issue. He clearly just wanted to be of help. So, I said yes, and followed him.

Non-Muslims, like me, who wanted to stay on to experience the prayers, were ushered into a large praying room. The enormous carpet that covered the floor was strategically marked for individuals to kneel to pray side by side, with all the spaces facing Mecca. The visitors sat on a few lines of chairs at the back of the room laid out especially for us. A steady stream of men began to enter the room to take their places for prayer. The young man who had escorted me downstairs must have sensed I was out of my depth and sat with me to explain the prayers as they happened. Not that I understood the language as it is said in Arabic, the language of the Koran.

As prayer time ended, a young girl who had been one of the guides at the street corner earlier in the day sat down beside me.

"Can you tell me about the male/female segregation?" I asked her. "I'm intrigued."

She was a jolly English girl who had converted, and I learned from her that ladies are always in a separate room nearby. I asked her what the reason was – I already understood that it was a general practice to keep the sexes separate, but I wanted to hear her views on this issue.

"The praying room has spaces marked out on the carpet and the rows are close together, so I think it's best to be separate from the men," she explained. "Besides, I don't really want to kneel to pray on the carpet behind some big bloke's bum."
We both laughed at her honesty.

There was no real mystique there that day. It was a day I witnessed a different religion, that I knew a little of, in a building used especially for the faith. It was simply just different from my Christian church's praying standards.

I am not a convert to the Islamic faith; some have said I should be highly incensed that my life was dramatically changed by this religion. But all religions have good and bad press. A simple statement to make, I know. But we hear of religious conflicts daily on television news items, of different faiths fighting each other all around the world in the name of their own religion. I simply do not understand it. Is it so difficult to honour others' religious views, even if they do not correspond to one's own faith or understanding? Maybe some people can only accept what they are used to, nothing different, nothing more.

I left the mosque feeling lighter, with a clearer vision of the proceedings inside, and a clearer understanding of Islam, a religion based on love, understanding, and tolerance. I'm glad I visited.

**

Despite all the heartache, I still felt lucky to have met Angelo in the first place, under relatively unusual dating circumstances, so many years ago. Those adventures we had together were probably unlike any most other couples would ever experience in their entire lifetime together. I was glad I never missed the opportunity to do those things. I was simply saddened that what I thought could be a great working partnership did not run a longer course, and beyond sad that our love story did not play out the way we both originally intended.

He is still Mr Smiley Person to me, adored by everyone who meets him. We still have great love between us, even though our homes, religions, and social lives are now quite separate. We live in the same town, and we still talk often. He will always be on hand for me should I need his support, and I for him. But I have finally moved on.

ABOUT THE AUTHOR

Trevor the youngest of 4 children was born and raised in Crewe, Cheshire by his Scottish mother and his Welsh father.

From a very young age he performed in endless amateur productions, had a part time stage crew job for over a year at his local repertory theatre where he was offered his first professional acting work having never been to a drama school.

He has worked in most of the regional theatres in the United Kingdom and Ireland and toured everywhere with large scale productions of both musicals and drama. Was lucky to gain an Arts Council grant to study with a top vocal coach in London and gained another Arts Council Grant years later to study The Alexander Technique after he fell off the stage at the Kings Theatre Glasgow and injured himself. Ooops!

Regional productions he has appeared in include The Lady from the Sea, The Government Inspector, How to Succeed in Business Without Really Trying, Hamlet, The Frogs, Jesus Christ Superstar, Annie, Coriolanus, Company, Othello, Funny Thing Happened on the way to the Forum, A Little Night Music, Amadeus, and Side By Side By Sondheim.

In the West End, he appeared in the following lead productions: Happy as a Sandbag, Godspell, Streamers, Cancer, The Boyfriend, The Dirtiest Show in Town and East which transferred from the National Theatre.

He was directed by Christopher Biggins in London and the Off-Broadway production of Narnia, Methusalem at Bloomsbury Theatre London and A Midsummers Night's Dream in Barbados.

The late Clive Donner directed him in two international movies: Alfred the Great (M.G.M.) and Here we go Round the Mulberry Bush (United Artistes).

Over the past eight years he has been associated with adjudicating Drama Awards for the Brighton and Hove Art Council's annual drama theatre awards.

Still a keen gardener a skill he learned from helping his father tend the local vicarage garden.

He is represented by theatrical agent Lesley Duff at Diamond Management.

ACKNOWLEDGEMENTS

Gratitude and thanks go to Lord Michael Cashman who, without any question, helped me over an insurmountable problem in my life. Eternally grateful.

To the hugely talented Stephen Mear for dragging me back to theatre life after an extraordinary bleak period, my huge undying thanks and love.

To Caitlin Mellon who creatively advised and encouraged me to finish the final manuscript and helped me over many hurdles, I thank her most sincerely.

BIBLIOGRAPHY

Albery Theatre. Now Noel Coward Theatre, Charing Cross Rd, London
Alfred The Great. MGM movie. Book-James R Webb 1968
Annie. 1977 Music- Charles Strouse, Lyrics- Martin Charmin. Book- Thomas Meehan
Blood Brothers. 1983 Book Lyrics and music -Willy Russell
Christ and St Stevens, West 69th St New York NY 10023
Clive Donner. Film director 1926-2010
Jesus Christ Superstar. Music -Andrew Lloyd Webber. Lyrics - Tim Rice
Jose Carreras. Spanish operatic tenor.
Godspell. 1971 Music, lyrics -Stephen Schwartz / John-Michael Tebelak
Gerald Malcolm Durrel OBE (7 January 1925-30 January 1995) British naturalist, writer, zookeeper, conservationist, and television presenter.
Henry Scott Holland. Poem-Death is nothing at all.
How to Succeed in Business Without Really Trying. 2005 Music-Frank Loesser. Book-Abe Burrows/Jack Weinstock/ Willie Gilbert,
Love Me Do. The Beatles 1962
Lyceum Theatre, Heath St, Crewe. CW1 2DA
Mozart. Alleluia, Exsultate Jubilate 1773
Narnia. 1986 Based on book by C.S. Lewis. Music- Thomas Tierney. Lyrics- Ted Drachman. Book- Jules Tasca
Noises Off. Michael Frayn 1982
Polka Theatre 240 The Broadway London SW19 1SB
Royal Central School of Speech and Drama. Swiss Cottage, Eton Ave, Belsize Park, London NW3 3HY
Snoopy. 1988 Music- Larry Grossman. Lyrics- Hal Hackady. Book- Warren Lockhart, Arthur Whitelaw, Michael Grace
Suddenly Last Summer. Tennessee Williams
The Boyfriend. 1954. Music, lyrics, book- Sandy Wilson-
The Duchess Theatre, Catherine St, London WC2B 5LA
The Government Inspector. Book - Nikolai Gogol. Translation- Alistair Beaton
The Sound of Music. Music / lyrics - Oscar Hammerstein.

For the many young people, who suffered and were lost far too soon during the extraordinary Aids period, your memories live on, you will not be forgotten.